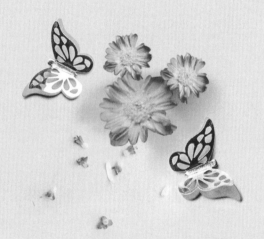

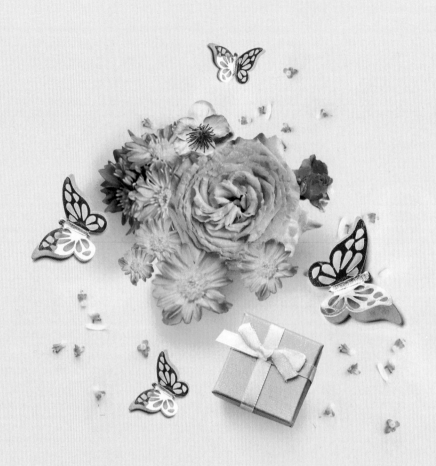

THE COMPLETE GUIDE TO
SELF CARE

Best Practices for a Healthier and Happier You

Kiki Ely

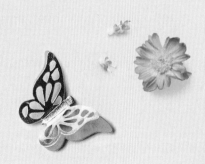

CHARTWELL
BOOKS

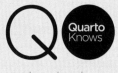

Brimming with creative inspiration, how-to projects, and useful information to enrich your everyday life, Quarto Knows is a favorite destination for those pursuing their interests and passions. Visit our site and dig deeper with our books into your area of interest: Quarto Creates, Quarto Cooks, Quarto Homes, Quarto Lives, Quarto Drives, Quarto Explores, Quarto Gifts, or Quarto Kids.

© 2020 Quarto Publishing Group USA Inc.

First published in 2020
by Chartwell Books,
an imprint of The Quarto Group

142 West 36th Street,
4th Floor
New York, NY 10018
USA

T (212) 779-4972
F (212) 779-6058

www.QuartoKnows.com

Chartwell Books titles are also available at discount for retail, wholesale, promotional, and bulk purchase. For details, contact the Special Sales Manager by email at specialsales@quarto.com or by mail at The Quarto Group, Attn: Special Sales Manager, 100 Cummings Center Suite 265D, Beverly, MA 01915, USA.

Library of Congress Cataloging-in-Publication Data

Names: Ely, Kiki, author.
Title: The complete guide to self-care : best practices for a healthier and happier you / Kiki Ely.
Description: New York, NY : Chartwell Books, an imprint of The Quarto Group, 2020.
| Includes bibliographical references. | Summary:
  "Self-care is far from selfish. Learn lots of new mantras, tips, tricks,
  and crafts to help balance out all the moving parts in your life with
  The Complete Guide to Self-Care"-- Provided by publisher.
Identifiers: LCCN 2019051272 (print) | LCCN 2019051273 (ebook) | ISBN
  9780785838302 (hardcover) | ISBN 9780760367964 (ebook)
Subjects: LCSH: Self-care, Health.
Classification: LCC RA776.95 .E49 2020 (print) | LCC RA776.95 (ebook) |
  DDC 613--dc23
LC record available at https://lccn.loc.gov/2019051272
LC ebook record available at https://lccn.loc.gov/2019051273

10 9 8 7 6 5 4 3 2 1

ISBN: 978-0-7858-3830-2

Publisher: Rage Kindelsperger
Creative Director: Laura Drew
Managing Editor: Cara Donaldson
Editor: Leeann Moreau
Book Design: Evelin Kasikov

Printed in Singapore COS022020

This book provides general information. It should not be relied upon as recommending or promoting any specific diagnosis or method of treatment for a particular condition, and it is not intended as a substitute for medical advice or for direct diagnosis and treatment of a medical condition by a qualified physician. Readers who have questions about a particular condition, possible treatments for that condition, or possible reactions from the condition or its treatment should consult a physician or other qualified healthcare professional.

*"An empty lantern
provides no light. Self-care
is the fuel that allows your
light to shine brightly."*

—UNKNOWN

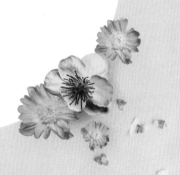

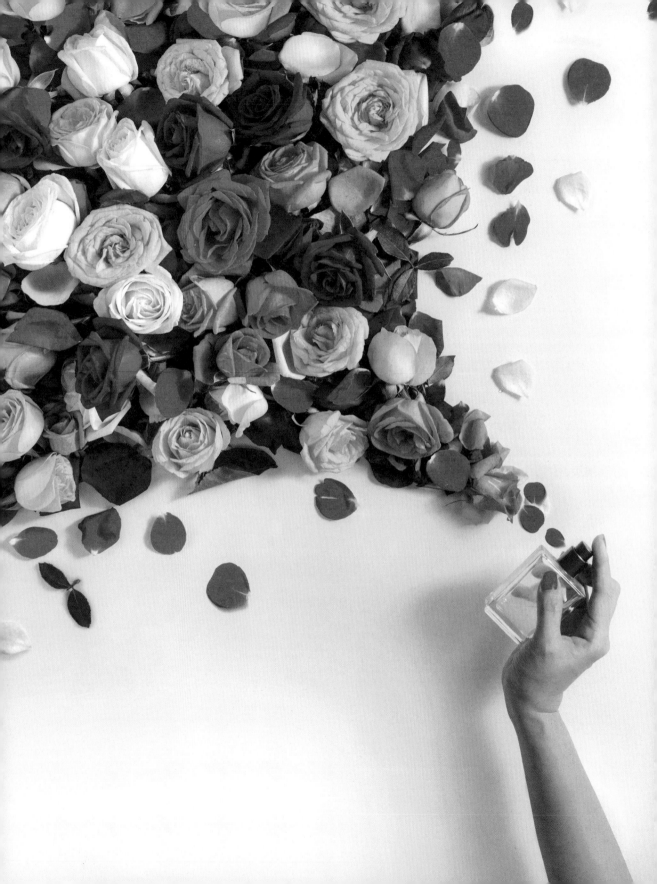

Contents

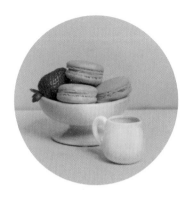

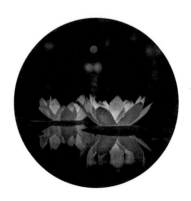

2
INTELLECTUAL SELF-CARE

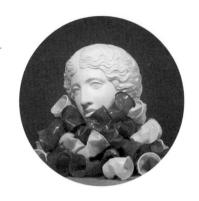

3
EMOTIONAL SELF-CARE

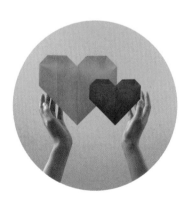

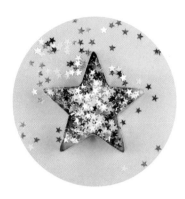

4

SPIRITUAL SELF-CARE

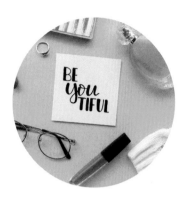

5

SOCIAL SELF-CARE

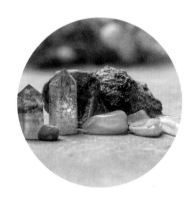

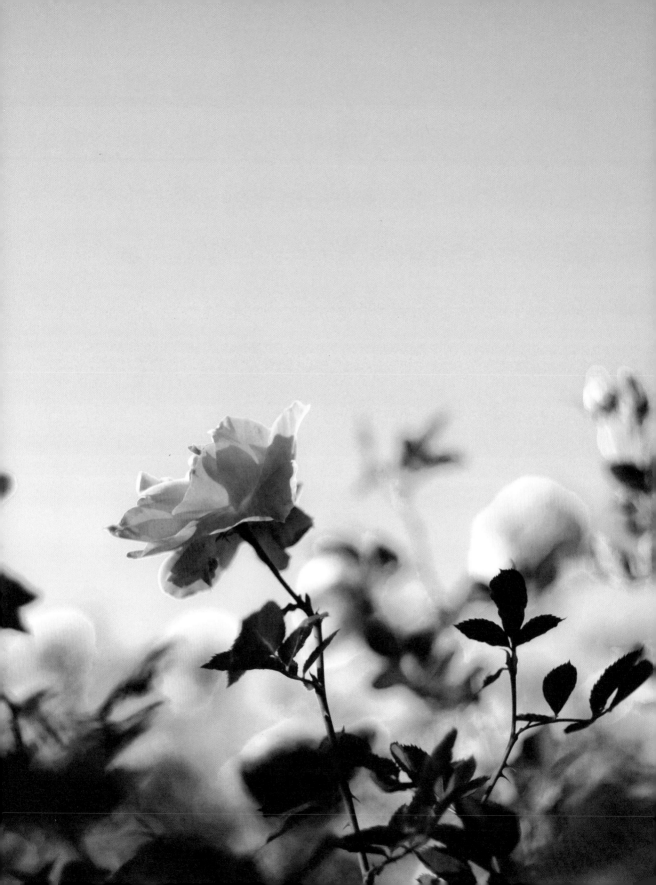

Introduction

You were put on this earth to live a radically fulfilling, purpose-driven, joyful life. You are worthy of this kind of life. You deserve to wake up each day with excitement coursing through your body and spirit in anticipation for what lies ahead.

_____

Unfortunately, this kind of life is elusive for many. In our distracting, fast-paced, demanding world, it can become easy to put yourself last. You may find yourself putting your needs at the bottom of your ever-growing to-do list. Maybe you actively prioritize the needs of everyone else above your own. Perhaps you're depleted at the end of the day, exhausted from trying to satisfy everyone else but yourself. Sound familiar?

Simply put, our modern world is riddled with modern illnesses. These illnesses have names like:

Overwhelm

Burnout

Low Self-Esteem

Anxiety

Loneliness

Lack of Motivation

Grief

Heartache

Feeling Lost

If you suffer from one of these modern afflictions, you're not alone. The good news is that you have it within your power to heal yourself and replace those painful feelings with:

Calm

Energy

Confidence

Focus

Introspection

Inspiration

Hope

Love

Purpose

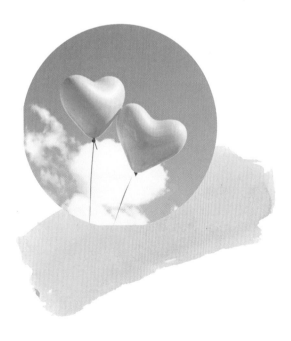

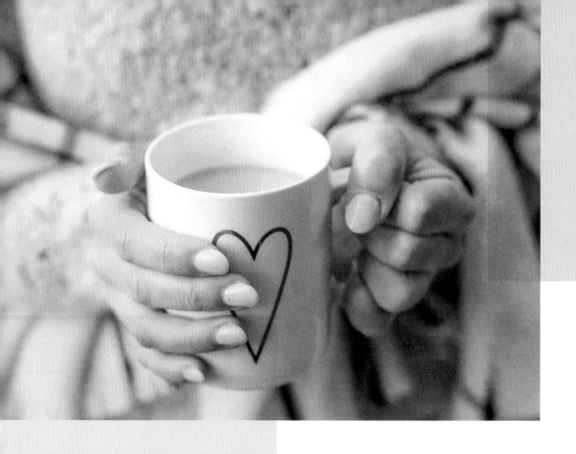

The antidote is self-care. This book is full of thoughtful advice, accessible exercises, healing rituals, and time-tested solutions to help you achieve the kind of inner peace and sense of self that leads to a happy, balanced, and stable life. Use this book as a guide to help you identify and fulfill your needs to lead the kind of life you've always wanted.

What is Self-Care?

Self-care is something you do to take care of your physical, intellectual, emotional, spiritual, or social health. It is done thoughtfully and with the intention of caring for yourself in order to increase happiness, focus, stability, joy, peace, feelings of gratitude, and self-love.

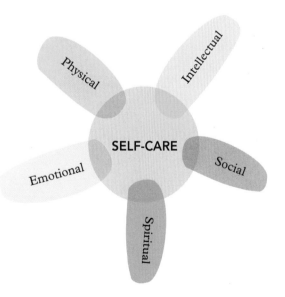

Why is Self-Care Important?

The world continues to move at a quickening pace—and this demand on your most valuable resource, time, is unsustainable. Self-care is a way to reclaim your power, recalibrate your body and mind, and establish your own natural pace. When you practice self-care, you can harness your own energy to make more intentional decisions. You'll also decrease anxiety, gain fulfillment, and attract more of what you truly seek into your life. It also increases confidence and helps you stay happy. As you love yourself and others, you will bring light into an otherwise chaotic, fast-paced world.

How to Use This Book

This book is meant to be used and shared in whatever way you see fit. Even though the official title is *The Complete Guide to Self-Care*, I want you to read it as:

> [*Insert Your Name Here*]'s
>
> Complete Guide to Self-Care.

Self-care is an individual journey, so there's no "right" or "wrong" way to use this book—its content is here to serve you in the best way for you. You can use this book in the following ways:

Read it from start to finish. This book was written in a way that it starts with basic self-care tenets that many people tend to overlook, like how to get a restful night of sleep or what proper nourishment looks like. It then moves on to internal elements of self-care that involve your mind and emotions. Next, it explores self-care spiritual exercises. The book culminates with how you can apply your new self-cared-for-self to the world around you.

Read it section by section. You can choose sections that are relevant to what you're going through now.

Maybe you've gone through heartbreak and you're drawn to emotional self-care. Perhaps you're seeking to gain a deeper awareness of yourself, so you might want to dive into intellectual self-care. Maybe you've always been curious about connecting to a higher energy and want to explore spiritual self-care. Or maybe you're looking to nurture your body in a more meaningful way and want to focus on physical self-care.

Pick one exercise from each section. If you want to dive right into self-care, you can "speed read" through and pick an exercise from each section to complete. You can then come back and read it in its entirety.

Do the exercises in the book with others. You can pick a few exercises a week to do with a group of friends or choose a section to read each month with your book club. Or work with one friend and hold each other accountable for completing the exercises and prioritizing self-care.

Use the book to benefit the greater whole. You can use this book as a guide for group retreat work. Or it can be incorporated into your workplace as company-wide suggested reading or for departments to read and discuss in reading circles.

Let your intuition guide you. Pick something by simply scanning the table of contents and see which section or sections jump out at you. Or open to a page and trust that its content is what you need to focus on in the present moment.

Whichever way you choose to use this book, I hope it brings you a step closer to happiness, a life you're passionate about, and true self-love.

Love (and lots of light),

KIKI
@blonderambitions
#thecompleteguidetoselfcare

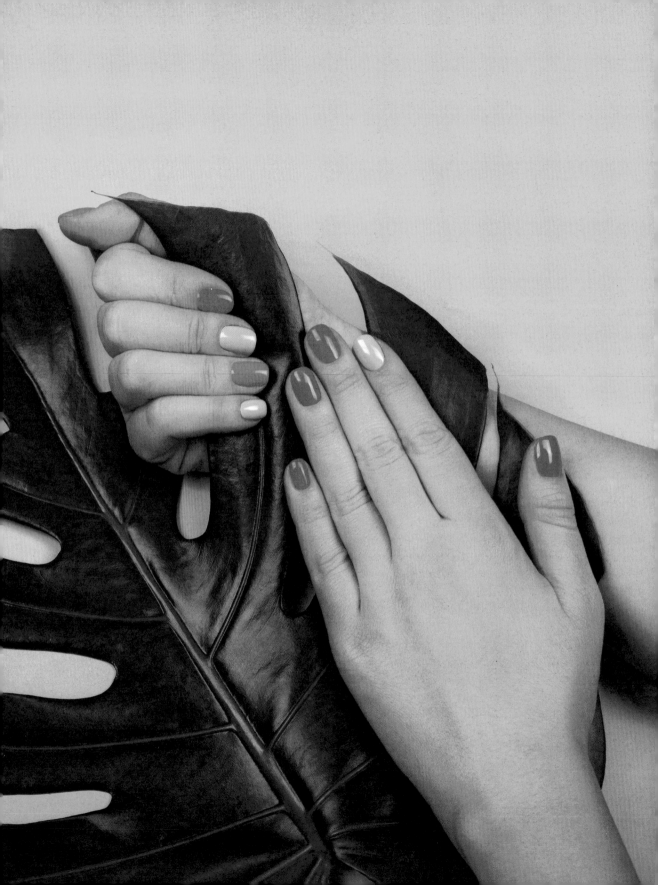

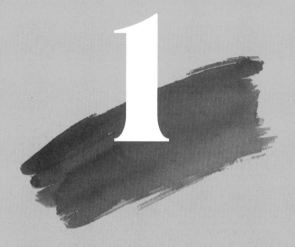

PHYSICAL SELF-CARE

"Your body is precious.
It is our vehicle for awakening.
Treat it with care."

—BUDDHA

Movement

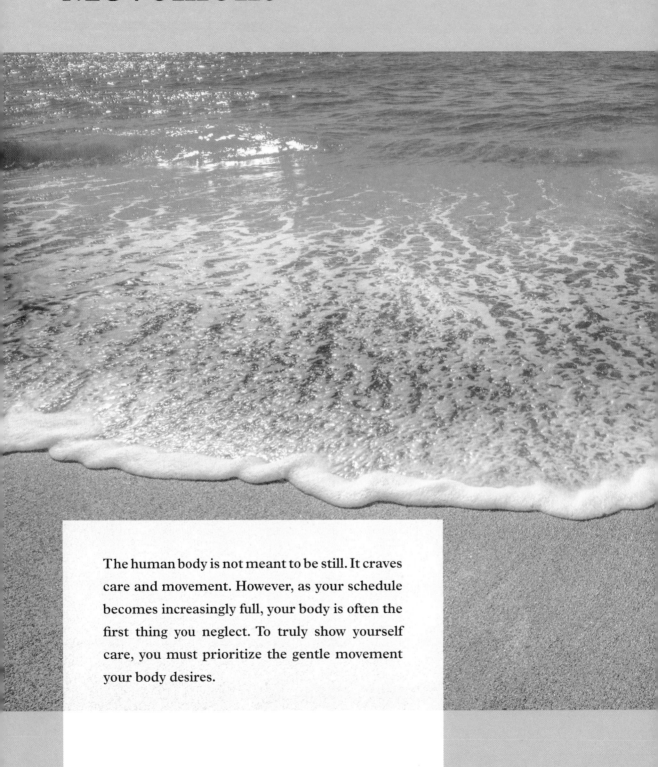

The human body is not meant to be still. It craves care and movement. However, as your schedule becomes increasingly full, your body is often the first thing you neglect. To truly show yourself care, you must prioritize the gentle movement your body desires.

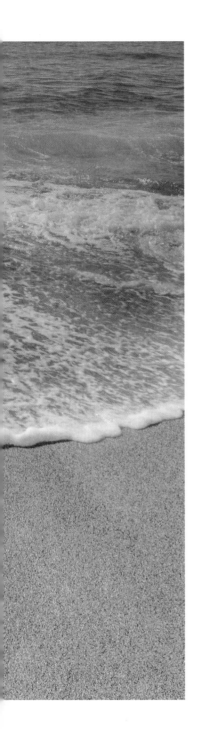

Benefits of Daily Movement

If you need motivation to get moving, as many people do, here are some of the incredible benefits that you can reap from just thirty minutes of movement a day:

———

Mood: The increase in endorphins and other mood-boosting brain chemicals can help increase happiness, decrease anxiety, and battle depression.

Energy: Movement increases the amount of oxygen and nutrients that get delivered throughout your body. This internal flow gives your heart and lungs more love, which makes them more efficient and increases your energy level.

Overall Health: An immediate benefit of exercise is that your immune system gets a boost. With consistent movement worked into your self-care routine, you can help prevent heart disease, lower blood pressure, fight depression and anxiety, prevent or manage cancer, combat arthritis, decrease chance of stroke, and reduce the risk of type 2 diabetes.

Weight Management: Daily movement can burn excess calories and keep your weight within a healthy range.

Self-Confidence: Movement connects you to your body and helps improve your physical self-image. This benefits your confidence and even your sex drive!

Better Sleep: As long as you don't exercise at night (which can make sleeping more difficult), movement during the day can help you fall asleep faster and stay asleep longer.

Yoga

Yoga is an ancient self-care practice that has been used for overall well-being for over 5,000 years. This section will focus on *asana*, the physical postures that increase stamina, strength, and are believed to purify the body.

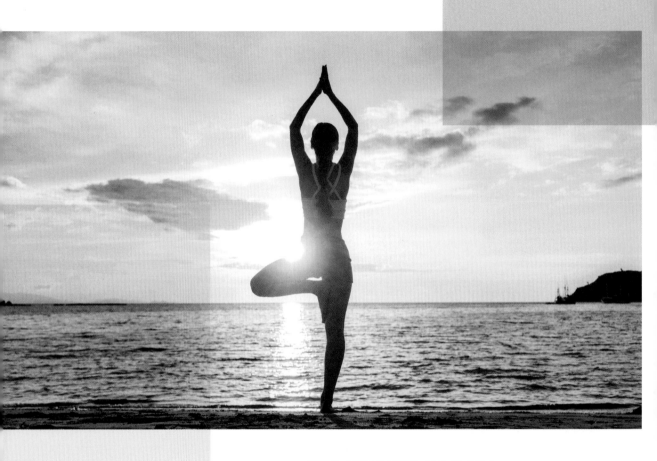

THE BENEFITS OF YOGA

The benefits of yoga extend far beyond physical fitness. Incorporating a yoga practice into your self-care routine also leads to clarity, focus, decreased stress and anxiety, increased sense of wellness, and both physical and emotional healing. Additionally, yoga provides the tangible benefits of better posture, balance, increased energy, more efficient digestion, and lubrication of your joints.

Three Basic Postures

For each of the following yoga poses, known as "postures," you'll want to focus on slow and measured breathing. This helps your mind and body relax and sends a soothing signal to your nervous system.

Mountain Pose

This standing pose is wonderful for relaxation, core strength, and posture. Stay in this foundational pose for one minute, breathing evenly.

STEP ONE: Keep your arms at your sides and your feet together.

STEP TWO: Press your feet evenly into the ground. This is known as "grounding."

STEP THREE: Press your tailbone forward so it's even with your spine. You should feel your thigh muscles activate.

STEP FOUR: Breathe in through your nose and extend your arms up above your head.

STEP FIVE: Breathe out through your mouth as you lower your arms to your sides. You should feel your shoulder blades push back.

Cat/Cow Pose

This pose gently engages your core and stretches out your back. If you are accustomed to sitting a lot in your daily life, this is a great way to elongate the spine, lengthen your abs, stretch your back, and fix posture issues. Repeat this cycle five times.

STEP ONE: Get down onto your hands and knees. Keep your hands under your shoulders and your knees under your hips to stay aligned. Keep your spine neutral. You may want to use a mat for comfort.

STEP TWO: As you inhale through your nose, engage your abs and imagine your spine being pulled toward the ceiling. Relax your neck and allow your chin to roll in toward your body. Your spine should be lifted, and your body should form an upward arc.

STEP THREE: Exhale fully out of your mouth while holding this position.

STEP FOUR: Inhale through your nose as you slowly push your belly button toward the floor, raising your head so your eyes can look forward and pressing your tailbone toward the ceiling.

STEP FIVE: Exhale completely while holding this position.

Tree Pose

This yoga pose helps with balance, focus, feeling centered, lengthening the spine, stabilizing the hips, as well as stretching the legs, groin, and buttocks. A wonderfully calming and meditative pose, it can help you feel strong, grounded, and "rooted" like a magnificent tree. Hold this position for thirty to sixty seconds and then repeat with the other leg.

STEP ONE: Stand with your legs shoulder-width apart.

STEP TWO: Balance on your left leg, gently lifting your right foot up to your inner left thigh.

STEP THREE: Bring the foot up along the inside of your thigh as high as you can but do not place it on your knee. If you can't bring the foot this high, rest it on your inner calf below your knee.

STEP FOUR: Make sure the toes of your right foot are pointing down to the floor and that the right knee is facing outward to open up your right hip.

STEP FIVE: Take a moment to get your balance. Keep your left hip above your left knee with your pelvis facing forward.

STEP SIX: Once you have your balance, bring your hands together in front of your chest. It should look like you are praying.

STEP SEVEN: To assist with balance and meditation, find a fixed spot on the wall or the floor to help you focus and stabilize.

STEP EIGHT: Inhale deeply through your nose and exhale slowly out your mouth while you hold the posture.

Walking

Walking is a low-impact, stress-relieving activity that anyone can incorporate into a daily routine. Walking can be done virtually anywhere and requires very little equipment to get started—all you need is a pair of comfortable shoes.

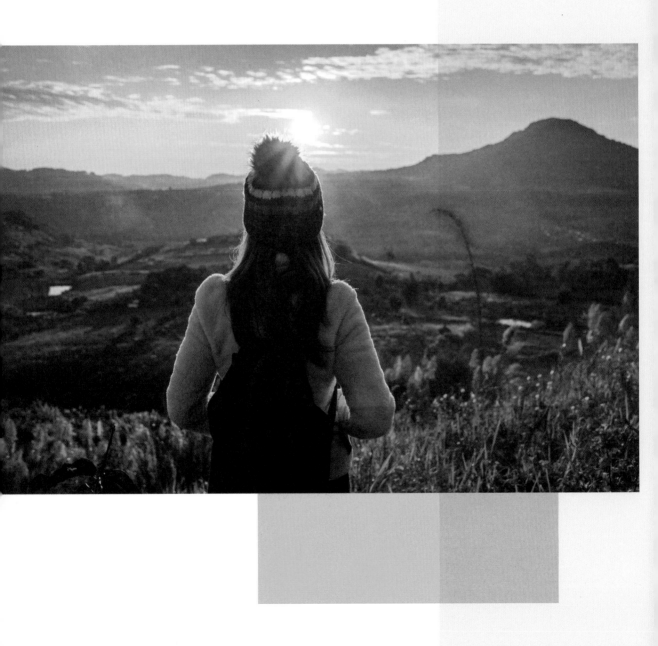

HOW TO GET IN YOUR STEPS

You should aim for 7,000–8,000 steps a day or 150 minutes of moderate activity a week. To meet this guideline and show yourself physical self-care, you could walk for thirty minutes, five times a week. Or you could break it up and sneak your steps in throughout the day. Bottom line: it doesn't matter how or when you do it as long as you do it.

Walking can easily turn into one of the most enjoyable parts of your daily routine. It is a perfect activity if you feel like you do not have enough time to exercise because it can fit into your day in seamless ways. Here are five ways to get yourself moving.

① **Take the Stairs:** It can be tempting to take the elevator, but it's better for your overall health if you tell yourself that the elevator is no longer an option. Walking up just two flights of stairs will awaken the muscles in your legs and get your heart pumping.

② **Park Across the Parking Lot:** It isn't practical (or even feasible) to walk everywhere, but if you must drive to a location, park all the way across the parking lot or at the top of the parking structure. This walk will get your body moving after sitting in the car.

③ **Efficient Walking:** Self-care can occur even in the middle of an overwhelmingly busy day. If you need to respond to emails, you can do so while walking on a treadmill set to 3 mph at a slight incline. This pace is slow enough that you won't be out of breath or too distracted to type, but fast enough to count as moderate activity. If you have phone calls to make (bonus self-care points if it's a conversation with a loved one), voicemails to listen to, podcasts to catch up on, or audio books to "read," invest in some Bluetooth headphones that connect to your smartphone and take a walk outside while you're checking other items off of your to-do list.

④ **Scheduled Walking Breaks:** To prioritize your physical self-care, get in thirty-minute walks every day. You can block out the thirty minutes in the following ways: one thirty-minute chunk, two fifteen-minute sessions, three ten-minute sessions, or six five-minute walks to break up each hour of your work day. Schedule these breaks into your calendar on your smartphone with an alert to hold you accountable. Want to walk at work? Bring comfortable shoes to change into. Plan to walk on the weekends? Set out on an early morning walk to start your day off on the right foot.

⑤ **Nature Walks:** If you want added benefits of increased relaxation, fresh air, vitamin D, and connection with nature, take your walk outside. You can stroll around your neighborhood, walk in a park, take a long beach walk at sunset, or try a new hiking trail. Getting outside and breaking out of your routine can provide you with such a sense of wonder and appreciation for beauty that you may not even notice that you're exercising.

Stretching

Stretching is a simple and calming way to incorporate physical self-care into your day and keep you connected to your body.

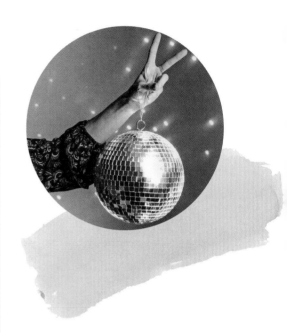

Adding a five-minute stretching routine to your day will increase your flexibility, improve your mobility, widen your range of motion, and help the blood flow to your muscles. It's a stress-relieving activity that can reduce headaches, assist your posture, help with body aches and pains, and protect you against future pain. Also, as you age your muscles are prone to feeling stiff and may even shorten. Stretching helps to maintain elasticity in your muscles, and it can also lengthen the muscles to keep your body limber.

The following routine works best when your muscles are warm. Before you start, briskly walk outside or in your home for a few minutes to get your blood flowing. If you don't have enough space to walk around, do some light jumping jacks for a minute or two. This routine utilizes *static stretching*, which involves holding a stretch comfortably for about thirty seconds; you can adjust this time period based on how you feel. When you're stretching, listen to your body—if something hurts, stop. Stretching can be a bit uncomfortable, but it should never be painful.

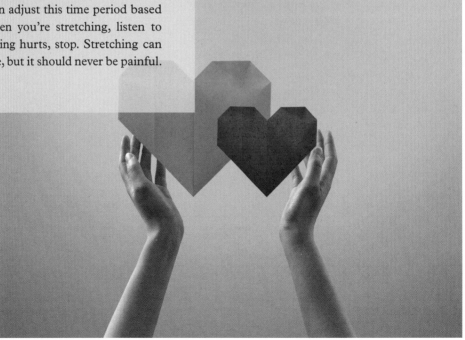

Daily Stretching Routine

Standing Hamstring Stretch

This stretch targets your hamstrings, glutes, and calves. It also provides gentle stretching for your neck and back.

STEP ONE: Stand comfortably with your feet shoulder width apart and knees slightly bent.

STEP TWO: Bend forward at your hips, while slowly lowering your upper body toward the floor.

STEP THREE: As you bend forward, keep your neck and shoulders relaxed as you breathe slowly.

STEP FOUR: Wrap your hands around the back of your legs to pull yourself closer to your legs without pushing to the point of pain while maintaining a microbend in your knees.

STEP FIVE: Hold for thirty seconds to two minutes.

STEP SIX: Bend your knees and slowly raise yourself back up to standing position.

Door Stretch

This helps open your chest and stretches your biceps.

STEP ONE: Find a door opening.

STEP TWO: Place your hands on either side of the doorjam.

STEP THREE: Lean forward until you feel a deep and comfortable stretch in your chest.

STEP FOUR: Hold for thirty to sixty seconds as you breathe easily.

Triceps Stretch

This stretch targets your triceps, but it has the added benefit of loosening the upper back, shoulders, and neck.

STEP ONE: Stand tall with your feet shoulder width apart and your knees slightly bent.

STEP TWO: Reach your right arm up into the air and bend your right elbow. Your right hand should be near the middle of your upper back.

STEP THREE: Use your left arm to gently push down on your right elbow to increase the stretch.

STEP FOUR: Hold for thirty to sixty seconds as you breathe easily.

STEP FIVE: Repeat with your left arm.

Knee-to-Chest Stretch

This is a relaxing stretch that can help loosen some commonly tight areas, including the hips, lower back, and hamstrings.

STEP ONE: Lie down with your arms by your sides and your legs outstretched.

STEP TWO: Keep your left leg extended and pull your right leg up to your chest with your knee bent.

STEP THREE: Breathe deeply and use your hands to pull your knee toward your chest.

STEP FOUR: Keep your lower back pressed into the ground to keep yourself supported.

STEP FIVE: Hold for thirty to sixty seconds as you breathe easily.

STEP SIX: Repeat with your other leg.

Butterfly Stretch

This is a great stretch for opening the hips, an area where many people store tension and have limited mobility. This stretch also benefits your back, thighs, and glutes.

STEP ONE: Sit on the floor comfortably with good posture.

STEP TWO: Bend your knees out to the side and press the soles of your feet together.

STEP THREE: Use your hands to gently push your knees down to increase the stretch.

STEP FOUR: If you're craving a deeper stretch, lean your body forward toward your feet.

STEP FIVE: Hold for thirty seconds to two minutes as you breathe easily.

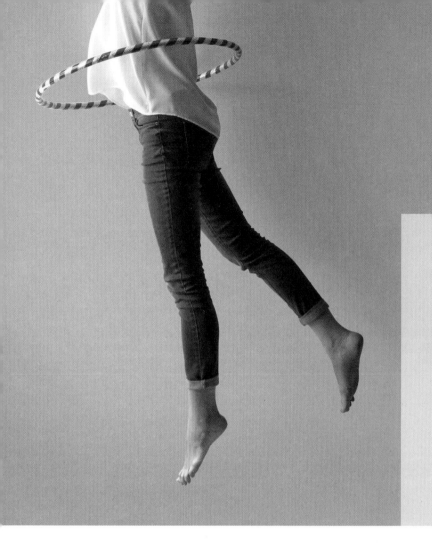

CONNECTING WITH YOUR BODY

The most important aspect of dance is connecting your spirit, instinct, and intuition with the physical movement of your body. So often we view our mind, spirit, and body as separate entities. But when you add music and movement, the three converge. In allowing yourself to connect fully, you're showing yourself love and care on multiple levels at once.

Dance

Dance signifies so many things: celebration, art, beauty, movement, human achievement, and our primal instinct to move to music. Dance has always been a part of the human experience.

Dancing is not about being good or bad, being on or off the beat, or having a certain body type. Dancing is about freedom, expression, and allowing your instincts to move through your physicality. In removing inhibitions or self-criticism while you dance, you're able to perform an act of self-acceptance and self-expression, which are both forms of self-care.

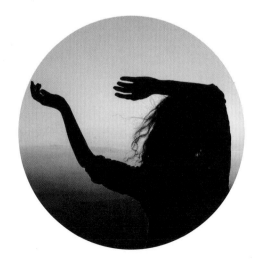

Intuitive Movement Exercise

The first step to being able to move intuitively is to remove the feeling of being self-conscious about your movement. If you love to dance and already move without inhibition, you may want to perform this exercise in front of a mirror. If this helps you love and appreciate your body and all the beautiful ways that it can move, then please incorporate a mirror into this exercise. If instead you feel a bit insecure when dancing, which is completely normal by the way, you should perform this exercise away from a mirror so that you aren't tempted to judge yourself.

STEP ONE: Find a song that you connect to and makes you want to move. Try to find something up-tempo that makes you feel energized.

STEP TWO: Play the song on "repeat" because you're going to be moving for about ten minutes.

STEP THREE: Start slowly by tapping your foot or snapping your fingers. Don't worry about being "on the beat." The only thing that matters is that you have your own beat.

STEP FOUR: Allow your shoulders and hips to join in the fun. Don't limit or censor your movements. Let your body go with the flow of the music.

STEP FIVE: Allow this physical freedom to spread to the rest of your body. Move in any way you see fit. You can jump, crouch, move your arms, roll your shoulders, crawl, kick, sway—do whatever your body wants to do. Close your eyes if it feels right.

STEP SIX: Notice how many different options you have when it comes to moving all your body parts: arms, legs, hips, back, hands, feet, neck, shoulders, and torso. Notice your fingers and toes too. Observe the endless combinations you can create with the movements of your body and explore a variety of combinations. This may feel strange because it's new, but keep going. You're expanding the relationship with your body.

STEP SEVEN: Continue this exercise for about ten minutes. When you're done dancing, take note of how you feel physically and mentally. Are you happier? Do you feel free? More beautiful? Energized? You'll notice how connecting to your body through movement can change your mind-set in only ten minutes.

Touch

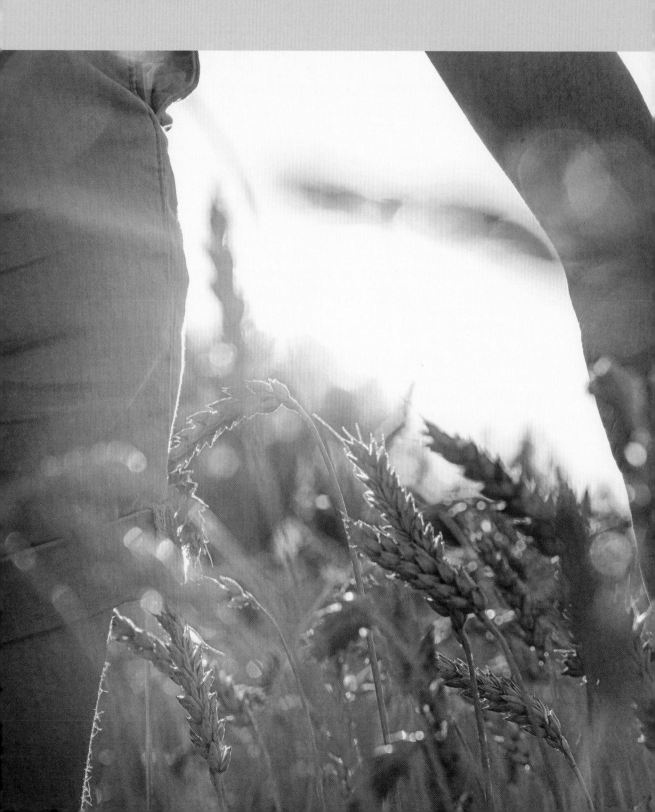

Your body is covered in nerve endings that allow you to fully sense what is around you. If you stop at any given moment to experience the sensation of touch—not just from another human being, but from all of the things that you encounter in the world—you might be surprised at all of the ways you experience the concept of *touch*.

For example, if you're reading this right now while sitting in a chair, you may stop and pause to notice the weight of your body touching the surface of the chair and the chair touching you back. If you're reading this book outside, you may notice the warmth of the sun's rays on your skin or a slight breeze in your hair. You may be wearing clothes that touch your body in certain spots, shoes that pinch your feet, or bracelets that knock against your wrist. If your hair is down, it may be brushing against your neck or shoulders. If you're legs are crossed, you might feel the points of contact between one leg and the other. In effect, you're constantly "touching" the world around you, but if you don't slow down enough to notice this experience, you'll miss out on a vital interaction with your surroundings.

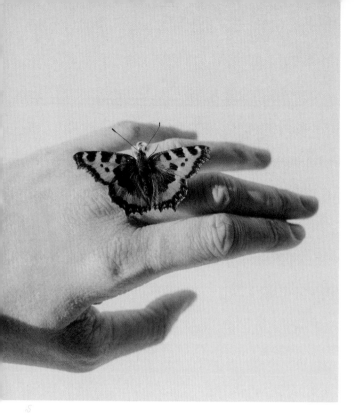

Why Touch and Your Senses are Important

To be fully present and able to care for yourself in the now, you must be aware of your surroundings. If you're not engaging your senses fully—touch being a primary sense—then you're essentially disconnected from the present moment and unable to fully participate in your life.

Self-awareness is a necessary form of self-care. You can't grow without this awareness, and the first step is being in tune with your senses. The sense of touch, your tactile exchange with the world, can unlock a whole new experience for you when you give it the attention it deserves.

Freeing Your Feet

Babies are barefoot when they take their first steps. Their feet *touch* the ground directly. And there's a scientific reason for this: shoes can negatively impact the natural development of the bones and muscles in a child's foot. Being barefoot and coming into contact with the ground in this early stage of life also aids the development of proprioception, which is the awareness or perception of the body's position and movement.

It's only with aging and the passing of time that you incorporate shoes into your daily routine. There are many obvious benefits to wearing shoes, namely comfort and keeping your feet safe. However, there are times when shoes are unnecessary and act as a block to the tactile connection with the ground beneath you.

BAREFOOT BENEFITS

There are many self-care benefits to walking barefoot. Here are a few:

- Walking barefoot lets you to move around the way you naturally would, which helps restore your gait.
- Bare feet can improve the strength and development of certain muscle groups, namely your legs, which act as a support for the lower back.
- Increased body awareness, posture, and balance results in more stable muscles and ligaments. [1]

Walking barefoot on any natural surface like grass, soil, or sand lets your body connect to the earth's natural charge, or electrons, a concept known as "earthing" or "grounding." There are many proven benefits of grounding, including:

- Decreased levels of pain
- Better sleep
- Reduction of stress
- Improved immune system
- A deeper connection with nature
- Ability to be more present

Grounding Exercise

STEP ONE: Find an outdoor area: grass, sand, soil, or anything safe and easy on your feet.

STEP TWO: Stand barefoot on the natural surface for five to ten minutes while breathing deeply.

STEP THREE: Walk barefoot on the ground for another five to ten minutes.

STEP FOUR: Try to incorporate getting your bare feet into nature and in contact with the ground at least three days a week.

Massage

A massage can feel luxurious and self-indulgent, and it should. Self-care is about recognizing your needs and then fulfilling them. Keeping this in mind, a massage is not so much a luxury as it is a self-care necessity.

BENEFITS OF MASSAGE

The benefits of massage span from physical benefits all the way to emotional and spiritual benefits. While you take the time to honor your body through intentional healing touch, you can reap the following benefits[2]:

• Reduced stress and anxiety

• Relief of muscle pain

• Soothing of digestive disorders

• Released tension in the body

• Sense of care and connection

• Relaxed mind and body

SELF-ADMINISTERED MASSAGE

You can participate in self-care by booking yourself a massage. Or you can administer massage on yourself in the comfort of your own home by using the following techniques.

EXERCISE

Foot Massage

Your feet carry your weight all day. Show yourself some care by giving your feet special attention to ease weary muscles and release tension.[3]

You'll need:

A tennis ball and a wall

STEP ONE: Stand near a wall so that you can lean on it for balance. With bare feet, stand on one foot and place the other foot on top of the tennis ball (if a tennis ball is too large for your foot, you can use a golf ball).

STEP TWO: Slowly roll the bottom of your foot on top of the ball, placing more weight onto your foot for more pressure.

STEP THREE: Focus on the arch of your foot, your heel, the ball of your foot, and your toes. Do this for one to two minutes, then switch to the other foot.

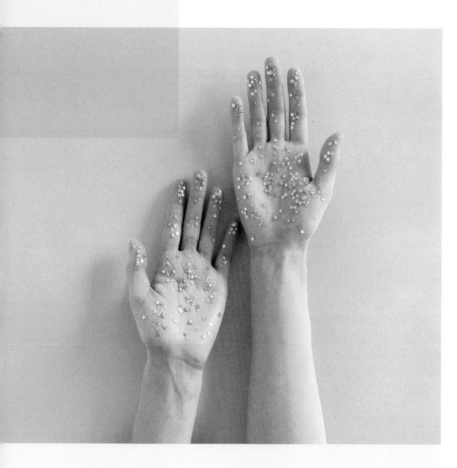

Calf Massage

Walking around or being on your feet all day can cause your calves to hold tension. Especially if you wear high heels, your calves could use a little extra care to soothe strained muscles.

You'll need:

A comfortable chair

STEP ONE: Sit in a chair with your bare feet placed gently on the ground. Lean forward and use your thumb to find your Achilles tendon. To locate your Achilles tendon, pinch your fingers on either side of the back of your ankle until you feel the strong, fibrous tissue that runs from your heel up the back of your calf muscles.

STEP TWO: Apply pressure and slowly rub the area until you feel tension release.

STEP THREE: Continue to do this up the back of your calf all the way up to the base of your knee until your calf feels relaxed.

STEP FOUR: Repeat the exercise on the other leg.

Hand Massage

Hands oftentimes get overlooked in a self-care massage regimen, but they're constantly working and deserve a break. It takes five minutes to give yourself a hand massage, and the results are immediate.

You'll need:

Lotion

STEP ONE: Apply a liberal amount of your favorite lotion onto your hands and rub them together until the lotion covers them.

STEP TWO: Take the thumb from one of your hands and use it to rub the palm of the other hand. Using one hand, pull each finger of the other hand gently away from the palm to lengthen and relax the fingers.

STEP THREE: Using one hand, push the other hand backwards and press to stretch your wrist.

STEP FOUR: Repeat on the other hand.

Neck Massage

Tension headaches, stress, and anxiety can all manifest as pain, stiffness, and soreness in your neck. Take a few minutes to help these muscles relax, which can diminish the stress and anxiety that caused them to tense up in the first place.

STEP ONE: Clasp your hands together behind your neck. Press your palms and fingers firmly but gently into your neck (on either side of your spine).

STEP TWO: Use your thumbs to rub out any kinks or knots by using a firm circular motion and then release your hands.

STEP THREE: Sit up straight and bring your left ear toward your left shoulder until you feel the right side of your neck stretch. Hold for thirty seconds.

STEP FOUR: Repeat on the right side of your neck.

Back Massage

The back acts as a primary support for your body and is where you may store emotional stress. It can be difficult to reach certain areas of your back on your own, so you'll need a tennis ball to help.

You'll need:

A tennis ball

STEP ONE: Place the tennis ball on the ground and lie down with your legs bent so the tennis ball is under your back.

STEP TWO: Using your arms and legs, gently move your body forward and backward on the tennis ball, pausing and lowering your body weight onto any areas of extreme tension.

STEP THREE: Do this for as long as you need.

Hip Release

Carrying tension in your hips and butt is so common because many people sit in a chair for most of the day. A sedentary lifestyle can lead to tight, closed hips. To remedy this, all you need is three minutes and a tennis ball.

You'll need:

A tennis ball

STEP ONE: Place the tennis ball on the ground and sit with it under your right butt cheek.

STEP TWO: Use your hands pressed against the ground to raise or lower your body and control the amount of weight on the tennis ball. Roll your butt cheek over the ball and pause anywhere there is tension.

STEP THREE: Repeat on the other side.

Eye Relaxation

Soothe eyes that are tired from staring at a screen.

STEP ONE: Rub your hands together until the friction has made them warm.

STEP TWO: Then place your hands gently cupped over each eye to allow the heat to relax your eyes.

STEP THREE: Repeat as many times as necessary until you feel your eyes get some relief.

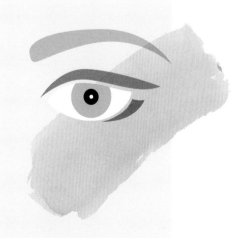

Comfort

It's natural to want to look good, but it all starts with feeling good. If your clothes don't fit, have scratchy fabrics, are poorly made, make you feel bad about your body, or don't fit your personality, you can change—or refresh—your wardrobe as an act of self-care.

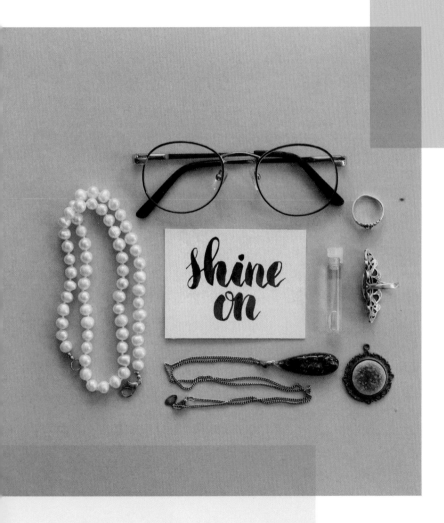

YOUR CLOTHING SHOULD FEEL GOOD

When purchasing a piece of clothing, ask yourself the following questions (if you answer "no" to any of them, you shouldn't buy it):

- Does the clothing fit me comfortably at my current weight?

- Does the fabric and all hooks/zippers/buttons/elastic feel good against my skin?

- Does this clothing fit my personality and lifestyle?

- Is this piece of clothing well-constructed?

- Can I move comfortably in this clothing?

Feel + Heal
Clothing Exercise

Imagine this: You walk to your closet and love every single item of clothing inside. Everything fits, is a representation of who you are, feels great on, and is something that you're proud to wear.

Sounds incredible, right? If this seems like an unreachable dream, think again. With some focus and commitment—all in the name of self-care—you can streamline your closet to become a stress-free space of self-expression that you love to visit.

Time Required:

A day or two, depending on the amount of clothing you own

Materials Needed:

Cardboard boxes

Full-length mirror

Matching hangers

(1) Label the cardboard boxes KEEP, DONATE, TAILOR, and TOSS.

(2) Take all clothing out of your closet and put it in a pile on the floor.

(3) Put on some upbeat music and try on the items of clothing one at a time in front of a full-length mirror.

(4) While you're wearing the clothing, ask yourself the following questions:

- Does it fit?
- Does it feel good?
- Is it my style?
- Is it well-constructed?
- Can I move comfortably?

(5) If you answered "no" to the question, "does it fit?" ask yourself if a slight alteration could make it fit comfortably and if it's worth spending the money. If the answer is "yes," put the item in the TAILOR box. If the answer is "no," move on to the next step.

(6) If you answered "no" to any of the questions above and went through step five, then it's time to decide if the item is in good enough condition to DONATE or if you should TOSS it. Place the item in the appropriate box.

(7) If you answered "yes" to all of the questions, then put the item in the KEEP box.

(8) Keep repeating this process for each item of clothing you own.

(9) When finished, place all items in the TOSS box in the trash.

(10) Bring all items in the TAILOR box to a tailor to have them altered.

(11) Bring all DONATE items to a homeless shelter, Goodwill, or local charity of your choice.

(12) Hang all KEEP items on matching hangers in an organized fashion in your closet.

(13) Repeat this exercise once a year to keep clutter and uncomfortable clothing at bay.

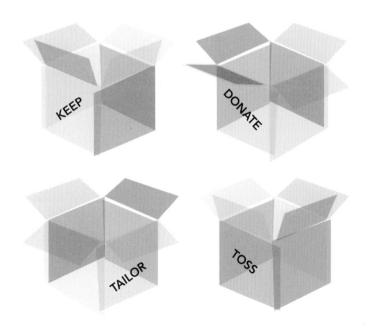

Sunlight

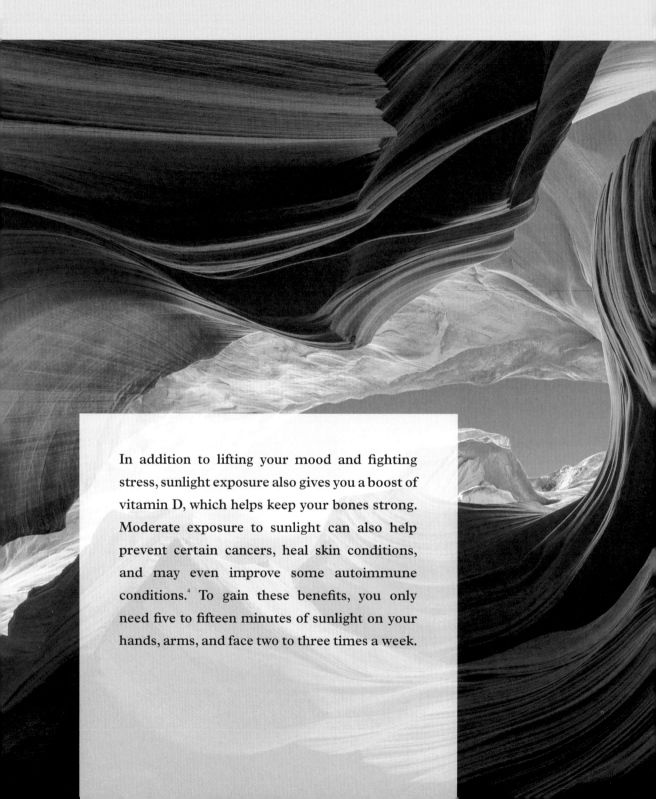

In addition to lifting your mood and fighting stress, sunlight exposure also gives you a boost of vitamin D, which helps keep your bones strong. Moderate exposure to sunlight can also help prevent certain cancers, heal skin conditions, and may even improve some autoimmune conditions.[4] To gain these benefits, you only need five to fifteen minutes of sunlight on your hands, arms, and face two to three times a week.

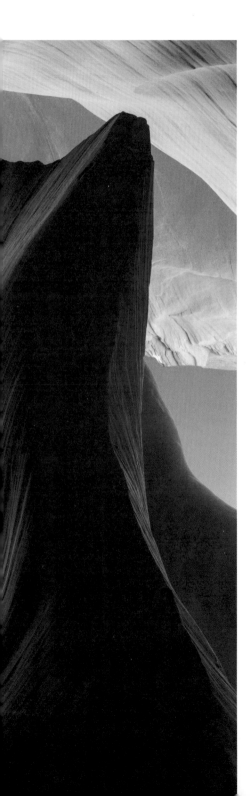

Soak up the Sun Exercise

Getting yourself outside first thing in the morning is a great way to start your day, set your circadian rhythm, boost your mood, and connect with your body.

Since early morning sunlight is gentle, it's generally safe to spend ten to fifteen minutes in the sun without sun protection in the morning. Commit to the following exercise to make spending time outside a habit.

STEP ONE: For five days in a row, preferably Monday through Friday, set your alarm for fifteen minutes earlier than usual.

STEP TWO: If you get up before the sun does, continue about your morning routine until the sun rises and then head outside. If you get up when the sun is already out, head outside right away.

STEP THREE: Find a comfortable position to sit and face the sun.

STEP FOUR: Allow yourself to breathe and stay in touch with your senses. How does the sun feel? How does your body feel? Can you hear any sounds?

STEP FIVE: Stay in this position for ten to fifteen minutes in silence, breathing slowly and taking in your surroundings.

STEP SIX: After five days of repeating this exercise, you should notice a positive shift in your mood, a more optimistic outlook, and lower stress levels. You may even feel more energized!

Being Present

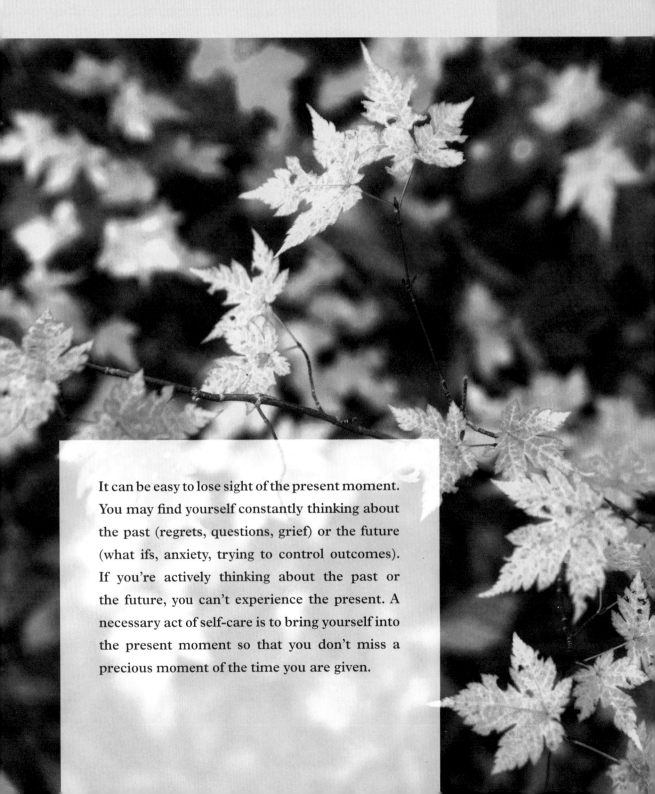

It can be easy to lose sight of the present moment. You may find yourself constantly thinking about the past (regrets, questions, grief) or the future (what ifs, anxiety, trying to control outcomes). If you're actively thinking about the past or the future, you can't experience the present. A necessary act of self-care is to bring yourself into the present moment so that you don't miss a precious moment of the time you are given.

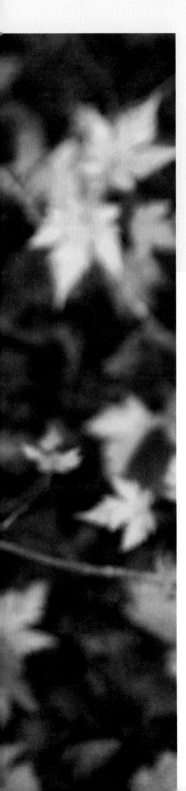

Five Senses Exercise

This simple exercise can be done anytime and anywhere to bring you firmly into the experience of your present moment. By recognizing your five senses, which are working all the time even if you don't notice them, you acknowledge your present experience. It is this acknowledgment that brings your consciousness back to here and now.

Ask yourself the following questions and respond in your mind. Or if you're somewhere private, you can say your answers out loud.

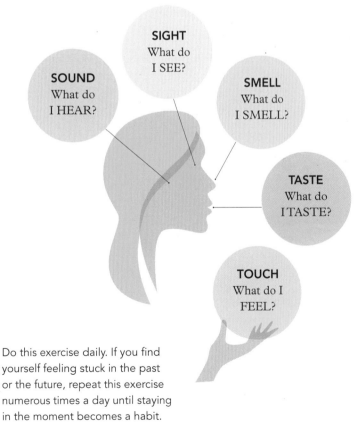

SIGHT
What do
I SEE?

SOUND
What do
I HEAR?

SMELL
What do
I SMELL?

TASTE
What do
I TASTE?

TOUCH
What do I
FEEL?

Do this exercise daily. If you find yourself feeling stuck in the past or the future, repeat this exercise numerous times a day until staying in the moment becomes a habit.

37

Hydration

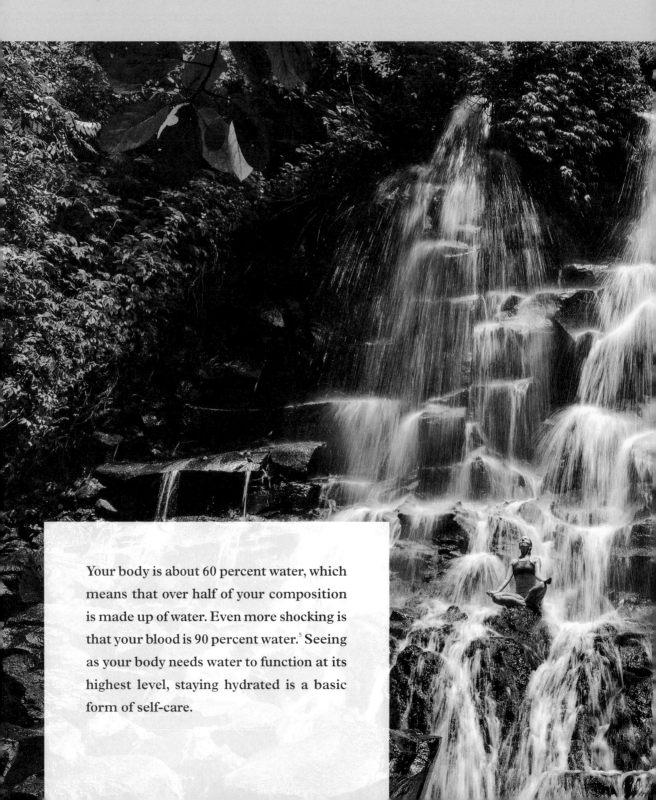

Your body is about 60 percent water, which means that over half of your composition is made up of water. Even more shocking is that your blood is 90 percent water.[5] Seeing as your body needs water to function at its highest level, staying hydrated is a basic form of self-care.

There are numerous benefits to drinking enough water every day. Here are a few key benefits:

———

- Keeps mouth clean and prevents tooth decay
- Assists with hydration of your joints, which are 80 percent water
- Prevents premature skin aging and can help skin look plump, dewy, and youthful
- Promotes weight loss
- Helps your body get rid of waste

Hydration Exercise

A simple formula for how much water you should consume daily is to take your weight and divide it in half to calculate the appropriate number of ounces of water you should drink. An example equation is: a 150-pound woman would divide her weight in half to get seventy-five. This means she should consume seventy-five ounces of water each day.

To make hydration a habit, do the following exercise every day for seven days. After you do this, staying hydrated will become a natural part of your routine.

You'll need:

An empty one-gallon water jug

A permanent marker

(1) Calculate the number of ounces of water you should be consuming daily.

(2) Put this amount of water into the water jug.

(3) Using a permanent marker, draw ten lines equally spaced from the bottom of the jug to the top of the water line.

(4) Set a timer on your phone to go off every hour for ten waking hours (starting right when you wake up).

(5) Each time the timer goes off, drink water until you get to the next marker.

(6) By the end of the day, you will have consumed the appropriate amount of water to stay fully hydrated!

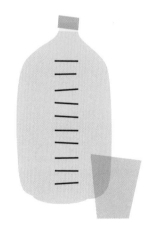

Healing Water

Drinking water is the easiest way to stay hydrated. The best way to consume water is at room temperature so that your body doesn't have to waste any energy heating it up.

If you're drinking water as soon as you wake up, which is highly recommended since you can become dehydrated while you're sleeping, try warm water with a squeeze of lemon and a teaspoon of apple cider vinegar. This is a very cleansing and alkalizing beverage that helps your body with digestion, boosts your metabolism, and cleanses the liver.

If you struggle to drink water because you find it boring (or don't like the taste), try infusing your water with fruit and herbs. All you need is a water infuser, which is affordable and can be purchased online. Try infusing your water with some of the following combinations:

- Watermelon and mint
- Peach and sage
- Strawberry and basil
- Lemon and mint
- Lemon, lime, and orange
- Grapefruit and mint

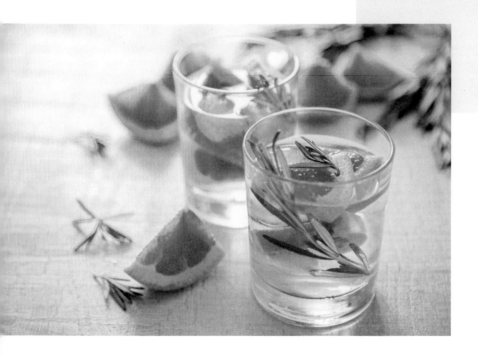

Healing Beverages

You can get hydrating, detoxifying, and healing benefits from other beverages besides water. Try incorporating a sweet and spicy celery juice into your morning routine, refreshing iced sun tea throughout the day, and sleep-inducing golden milk at night.

Sweet + Spicy Celery Juice

This juice tastes like a slightly spicy lemonade. Can't handle the heat? Simply omit the ginger.

You'll need:

A juicer

Ingredients:

A bunch of celery (6 large stalks)

Half a lemon

3 medium apples

3 teaspoons fresh minced ginger

Directions:

(1) Put all ingredients into the juicer. Drink first thing in the morning on an empty stomach.

TIP!

If you want the juice to be sweeter, simply add another apple. Or if you like it tart, use a whole lemon.

Sun Tea

Caffeine is acidic, dehydrating, exhausts the liver, and increases cortisol. So, non-caffeinated teas are a great (and healthy!) alternative that helps decrease your caffeine intake. An easy way to brew your favorite tea is by using sunlight.

You'll need:

A tea infuser

A large glass jar with a glass lid

Ingredients:

Non-caffeinated, loose leaf tea (try peppermint, vanilla, or something fruity like mango)

Directions:

(1) Fill the tea infuser with loose leaf tea.

(2) Fill the glass jar with purified water.

(3) Place the tea infuser in the water.

(4) Put the lid on the glass jar and put on a flat surface outside in direct sunlight.

(5) Leave in the sun for three to five hours.

(6) You can now enjoy your tea! Pour over ice for a refreshing drink. You can keep it in the fridge for two days.

Golden Milk

This soothing beverage is a traditional Indian drink that has been touted for its anti-inflammatory, digestive healing properties.

You'll need:

Saucepan

Stove

Your favorite mug

Ingredients:

2 cups (480g) milk (or a milk substitute like almond milk or coconut milk)

1½ teaspoons turmeric powder

½ teaspoon powdered ginger

1 tablespoon coconut oil

Pinch of black pepper

Directions:

(1) Put ingredients in a saucepan over medium heat and stir. Remove from heat when liquid begins to simmer.

(2) Transfer liquid into your favorite mug and enjoy while warm.

TIP!

If you want your milk to be sweet, add a little bit of honey or maple syrup.

Nourishment

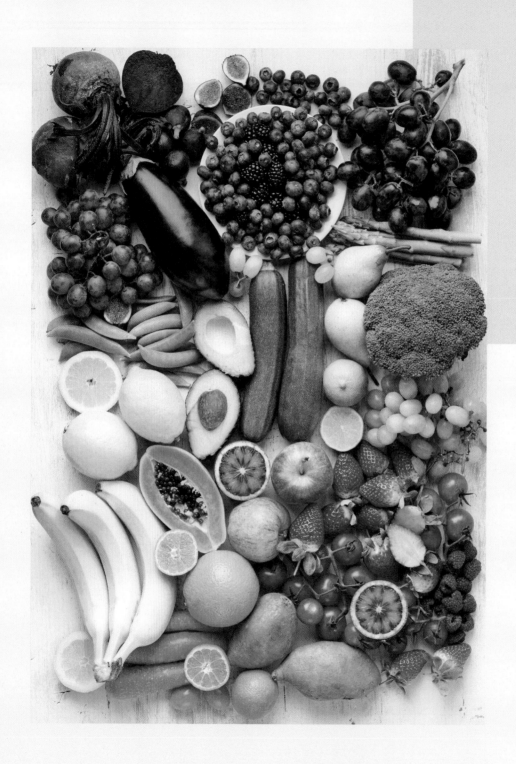

A properly nourished body is a properly loved body. Taking time to feed your body when it's hungry with nutrient-rich, healthy, whole foods is such an important part of self-care. When you nourish your body, you're taking care of yourself in a vital way. True health starts from the inside out.

Intuitive Eating: The Guiltless Diet

As babies, we automatically intuitively eat: we eat when we're hungry and stop when we're satisfied. As we grow, we begin to eat for other reasons: emotional comfort, boredom, addictive eating, cravings. A major form of self-care is getting back in touch with your body and recognizing the signs it gives you to eat when you're genuinely hungry and stop before you feel overly full.

But to get to this point, you first need to distinguish between physical hunger and emotional hunger.[6] Physical hunger is exactly what it sounds like. Your body gives you signs—such as low energy, hunger pain, a growling stomach, or irritability—which remind you that it's time to refuel. Emotional hunger is eating for any other reason besides physical hunger.

To truly show your body love and care, you need to get back in touch with physical hunger. Check in with yourself about once an hour and ask yourself, "Am I hungry? Is there a physical sign of hunger?" If you are experiencing physical hunger, gauge whether the hunger constitutes the need for a meal (oftentimes cued by a growling stomach or hunger pains) or if you need a snack (feelings of low energy or irritability). If you're unsure whether you are experiencing physical hunger, have a glass of water (sometimes craving food is simply a sign of dehydration) and check back in with yourself twenty minutes later. At that time, if you're not experiencing physical hunger, do not eat.

If it is time to eat, you should focus on two things:

① **Chewing:** Chew each bite thirty times. This helps break down the food so your body can easily access its nutrients. It also aids in digestion and gives your body time to recognize when it reaches a point of feeling full.

② **Conscious Eating:** Be present while you eat. Choose a peaceful location to enjoy and savor your meal. Taste each bite. Enjoy the experience. This also helps you take note of whether or not you're satiated.

This mentality connects you to your body and repairs—or enhances—your relationship with food. When you listen to the cues your body gives you, you're taking care of yourself.

HOW TO STOCK YOUR KITCHEN
WITH HEALTHY STAPLES

You'll be more apt to make healthy choices if you give yourself plenty of healthy options. Choosing to consciously nourish your body is an act of self-care that can impact your health, your mood, and your appearance.

Next time you go grocery shopping or to the local farmer's market, try to remember your ABCs and to "shop the rainbow."

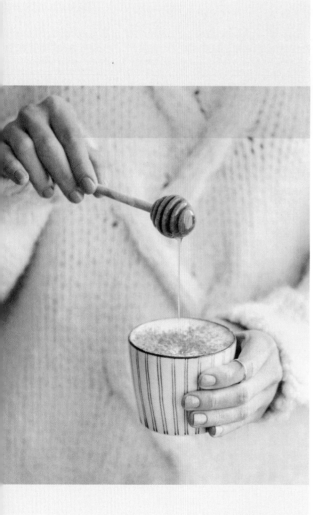

ABC SHOPPING

The concept of ABC shopping is simple: you should leave the store with apples and/or avocados, bananas, and cucumbers. The health benefits of these foods are incredible; they satisfy hunger and provide great nourishment.

- **Apples**: This high-fiber food also contains antioxidants that help improve brain health and lower cholesterol. They're also full of vitamins C and B-complex and are low in calories.[7]

- **Avocados**: This highly nutritious fruit contains twenty different vitamins and minerals. It is packed with fiber and potassium, has lots of monounsaturated fatty acids (great for your heart!), and can help lower your cholesterol.[8]

- **Bananas**: This easily portable fruit is a filling snack. It's full of fiber, vitamin C, vitamin B6, and potassium. It also contains prebiotics, which are great for your digestive system.[9]

- **Cucumber**: This low-calorie food makes a perfect snack or crunchy addition to any sandwich or salad. Snacking on cucumbers helps keep you hydrated and aids in weight loss—and they're packed with antioxidants.[10]

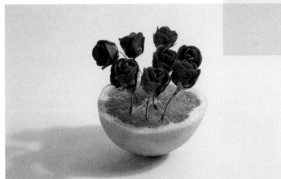

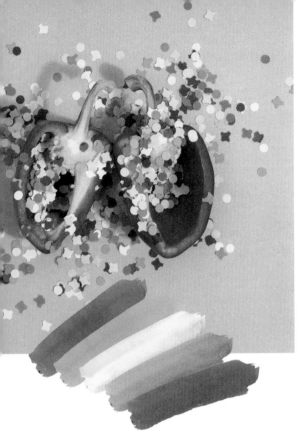

SNACKS

It's important to keep your kitchen stocked with healthy snacks and staples so that you can make thoughtful decisions when fueling your body. This concious investment in quality food is also a caring investment in your body.

- **Activated Walnuts:** Soaked in water and salt so that they are easier to digest, these are full of omega-3 fatty acids to help stimulate the brain and nervous system. Walnuts are also very filling!

- **Dehydrated Fruit:** This type of fruit can satisfy your sweet tooth. Mix some fruit with raw nuts if you need a heartier snack.

- **Dates:** They're known as "nature's candy" for a reason. One date after dinner can stave off your craving for a heavy dessert.

- **Nut Butters:** Almond butter and cashew butter are delicious, filling, and versatile. You can use them to make a sandwich, spread them on a banana, or just eat them straight from the jar.

- **Seeds:** This high-protein snack is very satisfying. Pumpkin seeds, sunflower seeds, and chia seeds are all great options.

- **Popcorn:** This easy-to-make snack can be a healthy option if you skip the butter. Try adding cinnamon, spices, or red pepper flakes to enhance the flavor.

- **Roasted Chickpeas:** This crunchy snack is delicious and full of protein.

RAINBOW SHOPPING

When you buy food, you should leave with something of every color of the rainbow. Red, orange, and yellow foods are known to have antioxidant benefits because they have carotenoids. Green vegetables tend to be high in vitamins A, C, and K. As far as blue and purple foods go, the darker the fruit or vegetables, the higher the antioxidant level. This ensures that you have a variety and are getting a wide array of nutrients and vitamins necessary for a balanced diet.

- **Red:** Apples, bell peppers, strawberries
- **Orange:** Carrots, bell peppers, oranges
- **Yellow:** Bananas, lemons, pineapple
- **Green:** Broccoli, kale, lettuce, spinach, herbs
- **Blue/Purple:** Blueberries, eggplant, plums, boysenberries, cabbage

Meal Preparation

Life has a way of getting unexpectedly busy—so you can stay a step ahead by preparing your meals in advance. This is a beautiful way to show yourself care because you'll have delicious and nourishing meals waiting for you regardless of how little time you have. There are endless meal prep ideas online, so take some time to research, prepare foods, and plan your meals ahead of time. In the meantime, here's a sample menu that will give you three days' worth of meals with a prep time of only thirty minutes.

RECIPE

BREAKFAST

Coconut Yogurt with Granola and Blueberries

You'll need:

1 16-oz mason jar

Paper towel

Elastic band

3 8-oz mason jars

Ingredients:

1 14-oz can full-fat coconut milk

3 strong probiotic capsules
(at least 25 billion CFU with no prebiotics or enzymes)

3 cups blueberries

4 ½ cups your favorite granola

How to make coconut yogurt:

(1) Pour the coconut milk into the 16-oz jar.

(2) Open the three probiotic capsules and empty the contents into the jar.

(3) Stir well with a spoon.

(4) Cover jar with a paper towel. Secure with an elastic band.

(5) Let rest for 24-48 hours, then put a lid on the jar and transfer the jar to the refrigerator.

How to make the parfait:

(1) Fill each of the 8-oz jars about halfway with the yogurt.

(2) Place 1 cup blueberries on top of the yogurt in each jar. The layer of blueberries between the yogurt and the granola keeps the granola from getting soft.

(3) Add 1 ½ cups granola on top to the blueberries in each of the jars.

(4) Store jars in refrigerator and eat within three days.

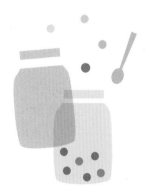

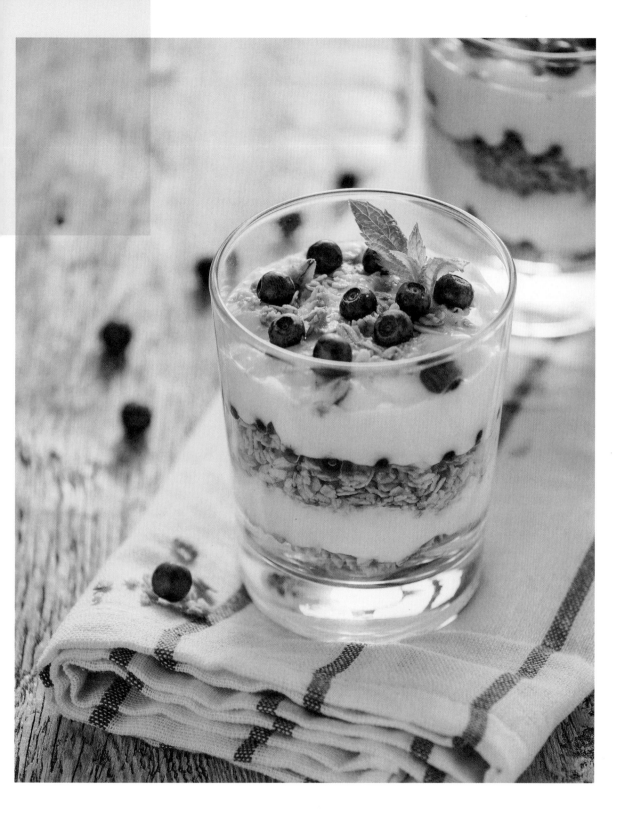

LUNCH

Salad in a Jar

You'll need:

3 16-oz mason jars

Ingredients:

6-8 tbsp dressing of your choice

3-6 handfuls of your choice of crunchy vegetables (carrot, celery, cucumber, onion)

3-6 handfuls of your choice of fresh vegetables (avocado, corn, fresh peas, tomatoes)

3 handful protein of your choice (beans, tofu, nuts, meat, poultry)

24 oz (660g) greens of your choice (romaine, arugula, kale, spinach, cabbage)

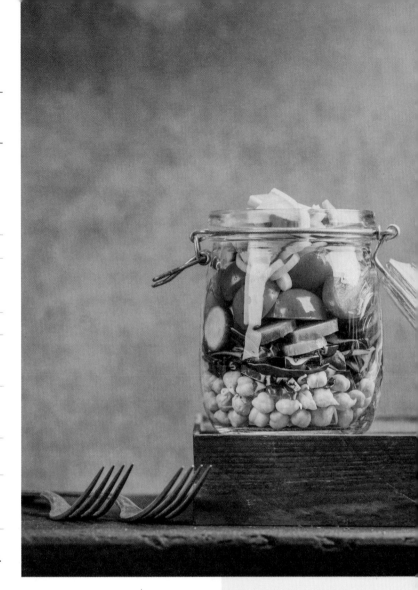

(1) Wash and chop your vegetables.

(2) Put 2-4 tbsp of dressing in the bottom the glass jars.

(3) Add 1-3 handfuls of the least permeable ingredients to the jars first (carrots, whole tomatoes, bell peppers, etc.) on top of the dressing layers. This is to keep the dressing separate from your layers of greens.

(4) Layer the remaining vegetables, distributing them evenly amongst the jars.

(5) Add 1 handful of protein to each of the jars.

(6) Add your greens to each jar, which should be about half of the jar's contents.

(7) Screw on lid and store in the refrigerator for up to three days. To eat, shake jar hard to incorporate the dressing and mix the ingredients. Eat the salad right out of the jar!

DINNER

Sheet Pan Fajitas

You'll need:

Sheet pan

3 microwave-safe
food storage containers

Ingredients:

1 ½ cups (278 g) brown rice

1 large red onion

3 bell peppers (any color you like)

½ lb (227 g) boneless, skinless
chicken breasts (omit chicken if
vegetarian or vegan)

3 tbsp olive oil

½ tbsp taco seasoning (to taste)

1 15-oz (439 g) can black beans

¾ cup (194 g) salsa of your choice

1. Make the brown rice.

2. Preheat oven to 425°F.

3. Cut the onions and peppers into strips and place on one half of the sheet pan.

4. Cut the chicken into thin strips and place on the other side of the sheet pan.

5. Drizzle olive oil over the chicken and vegetables. Sprinkle with taco seasoning.

6. Put in the oven for 25 minutes.

7. While the fajitas cook, put a layer of brown rice on the bottom of each food container.

8. Add a layer of black beans on top of the brown rice.

9. When the fajitas are done cooking, add a layer of vegetables and chicken on top of the black beans.

10. Top with salsa.

11. Place lid on the food container and store in the refrigerator for up to three days.

12. When you're ready to eat, heat in the microwave and enjoy.

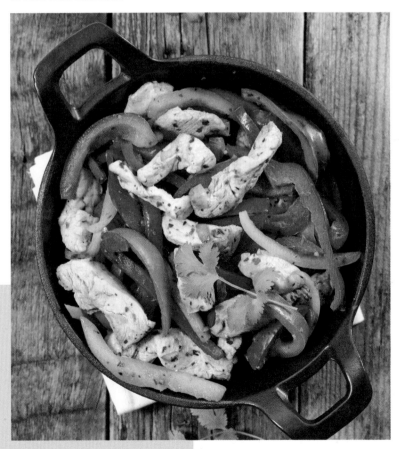

Beauty

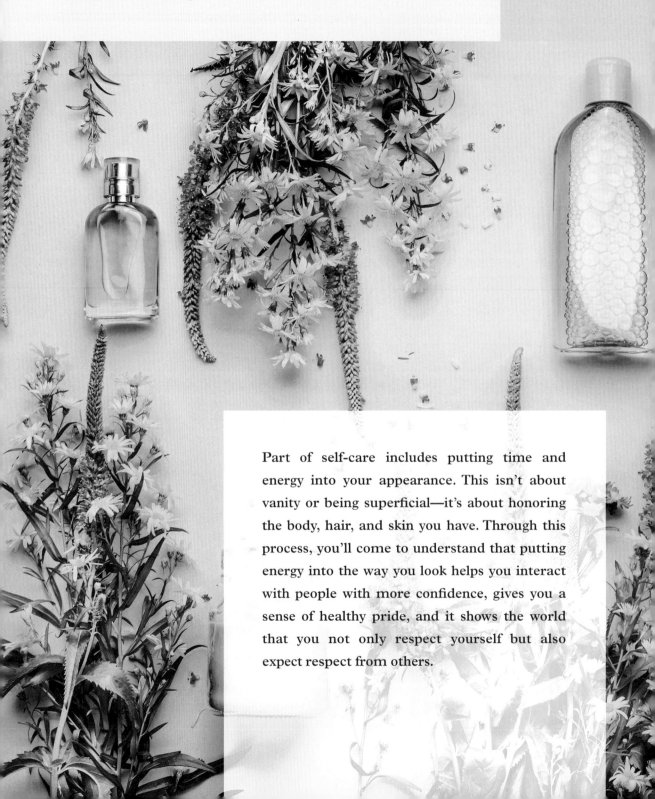

Part of self-care includes putting time and energy into your appearance. This isn't about vanity or being superficial—it's about honoring the body, hair, and skin you have. Through this process, you'll come to understand that putting energy into the way you look helps you interact with people with more confidence, gives you a sense of healthy pride, and it shows the world that you not only respect yourself but also expect respect from others.

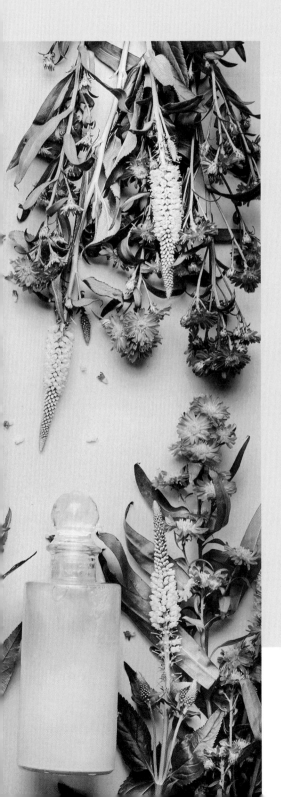

Beauty Ritual

A ritual is something that has a prescribed order and can be replicated, and it often has a soothing and empowering effect. You can create many different self-care rituals, with a beauty ritual being one of the easier to start with because it provides immediate visible benefits and only a bit of planning to implement.

———

But if creating your own beauty ritual seems a bit overwhelming at first, you can borrow the rituals and routines listed below. In time, you'll tweak them to make them your own, adding hints of your individuality until you've created your own bespoke beauty ritual.

Repetition and maintenance are the keys to turning something into a ritual. Commit to performing your specific ritual three times a week in the beginning. Then you can devote more time as you see fit until incorporating your ritual into your daily routine becomes second nature.

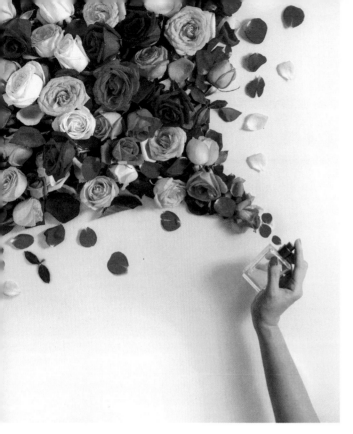

Oil Cleanse

Oil cleansing is when you use oil (yes, oil!) to wash your face. This helps break down makeup and remove impurities. This method has many benefits: it's hydrating, cleansing, soothing, less irritating than traditional cleansers. It also removes dirt, shrinks pores, and helps eradicate acne.

YOUR FIVE-MINUTE SKINCARE ROUTINE

Taking time to care for your skin has a myriad of benefits. It's soothing, calming, and rejuvenating (it slows the aging process). A daily skincare routine protects your skin from free radicals in the environment, eliminates toxins, and increases your radiance. Take five minutes every morning and then again at night to prioritize yourself and your skin. Besides, it's a relaxing—and refreshing—way to start and end your day.

This five-minute, five-step skincare routine includes simple, clean products that you can make at home. Plus, each step has a myriad of beauty and health benefits. Here's how to do a simple, five-step skincare routine.

RECIPE

Homemade Oil Cleanser

You'll need:

2 tsp coconut oil

1 tsp castor oil

How to Oil Cleanse:

Mix coconut oil and castor oil in your hands before using. The warmth will help turn cool coconut oil into a more workable liquid. Take your oil cleansing mixture and rub it in circular motions on your face (don't use water). You can use this oil cleanser to clean makeup right off your face or simply to nourish bare skin. Rub in circular motions for one to two minutes. Rinse with warm water and pat your face dry. Don't worry if there's excess oil cleanser on your skin because you'll remove it in the next step.

> **TIP!**
> Your oil cleanser can even be used on your eyes to break down waterproof makeup.

STEP TWO → Soap Cleanse

Cleansing with soap can be harsh on your skin, which is why you need to use a specific soap known as castile soap for this step in your skincare routine. Castile soap is powerful enough to remove the remaining oil residue after your oil cleansing—and even combat acne—but also gentle enough to not upset the pH of your skin. And it doesn't cause any irritation or strip your skin of its natural moisture.

STEP THREE → Tone

Toning is a quick step that removes any remaining residue, oil, cleansers, and makeup from your skin. It also helps keep your skin's pH balanced, minimizes the size of your pores, and increases your skin's natural radiance.

RECIPE

Homemade Soap Cleanser

You'll need:

Foaming dispenser

Liquid castile soap

Distilled water

Lavender essential oil

Lemon essential oil

Directions:

Fill a foaming dispenser one-eighth of the way with liquid castile soap. Add distilled water three-fourths of the way to the top. Add twenty drops of lavender essential oil and ten drops of lemon essential oil. Gently tip dispenser back and forth to incorporate the ingredients.

How to Soap Cleanse:

Splash face with water. Distribute 2–4 pumps of foaming soap cleanser into your hands. Rub the cleanser all over your face in circular motions. Rinse with warm water and pat your face dry.

RECIPE

Homemade Toner

You'll need:

Amber glass jar

Witch hazel

Rose water

How to Tone:

Fill the amber glass jar a quarter of the way full with witch hazel. Then fill the rest of the jar with rose water. Saturate a cotton ball with the toner and run the cotton ball all over your face.

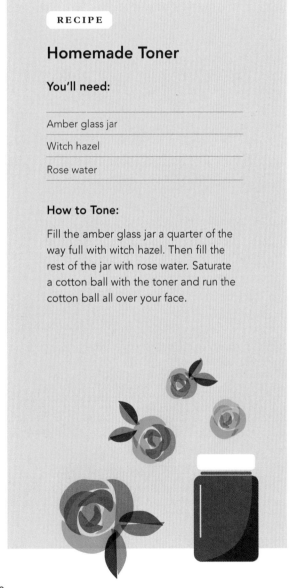

STEP FOUR → Facial Oil Moisturizer

Facial oil hydrates your skin by locking in moisture and helps combat fine lines and wrinkles. It also adds an extra glow to your complexion, can decrease dark spots, even out your skin tone, and reduce the appearance of dark circles under your eyes.

STEP FIVE → Facial Roller

Facial rollers are an ancient beauty tool that have been used in China since the seventeenth century.[11] You can buy a facial roller online or at a local beauty store. It has a large rolling end (for the forehead, cheeks, jaw, and neck) and a small rolling end for around the eyes and around the nose.

Facial rolling is a soothing way to end your ritual that helps relax tension in your face and promotes lymphatic drainage (i.e., it helps combat puffiness and gets rid of toxins). It can also further define your cheekbones and jawline, clear your sinuses, fight signs of aging, and reduce under-eye circles. Whether this last step is part of your morning or nightly skincare routine, the facial roller allows products to seep deeper into your skin for a makeup look that will last all day or a penetrating nighttime moisturizing remedy.

RECIPE

Homemade Facial Oil

You'll need:

Amber glass bottle with a dropper lid

Macadamia nut oil

Kukui nut oil

Argan oil

Jojoba oil

Rosehip oil

How to Moisturize with Oil:

Fill the amber glass bottle with equal amounts of each oil. Put the dropper lid back on the bottle and shake well to incorporate the oils. Take the dropper of oil and pour it onto the palm of your hand. Rub your hands together to warm the oil. Press the oil onto your face.

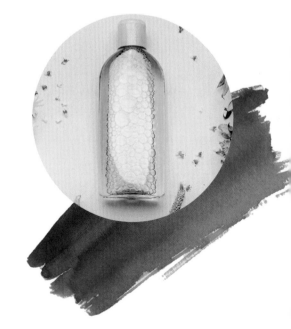

Facial Rolling

(1) Using the large side of a facial roller, start at your chin and roll upward along your jawline up to your ear. Do this ten times on each side.[12]

(2) Using the large side of the facial roller, start at the side of your nose and roll outward to your ear. Do this ten times on each side.

(3) Using the small side of the facial roller, close your eyes and start at the inner corner of your eye. Roll gently across your upper eye area out toward the temples. Do this ten times on each side.

(4) Using the large side of the facial roller, place the roller on your eyebrow and roll outward to your temple. Do this ten times on each side.

(5) Using the large side of the facial roller, move across your forehead rolling from your eyebrows upward toward your hairline. Do this across your entire forehead five times.

(6) Using the large side of the facial roller, start at the middle of your forehead and roll outward toward your temples. Do this on each side five times.

(7) Using the small side of the facial roller, start under your eye and run downward along the sides of your nose. Do this on each side five times.

(8) Using the large side of the facial roller, start at your chin and roll up along your jawbone ending at your ear. Do this on each side five times.

(9) Using the large side of the facial roller, gently roll from your jawline down your neck. Do this ten times on each side to assist with lymphatic drainage.

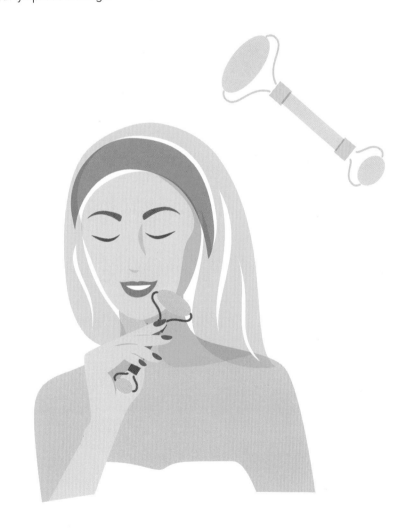

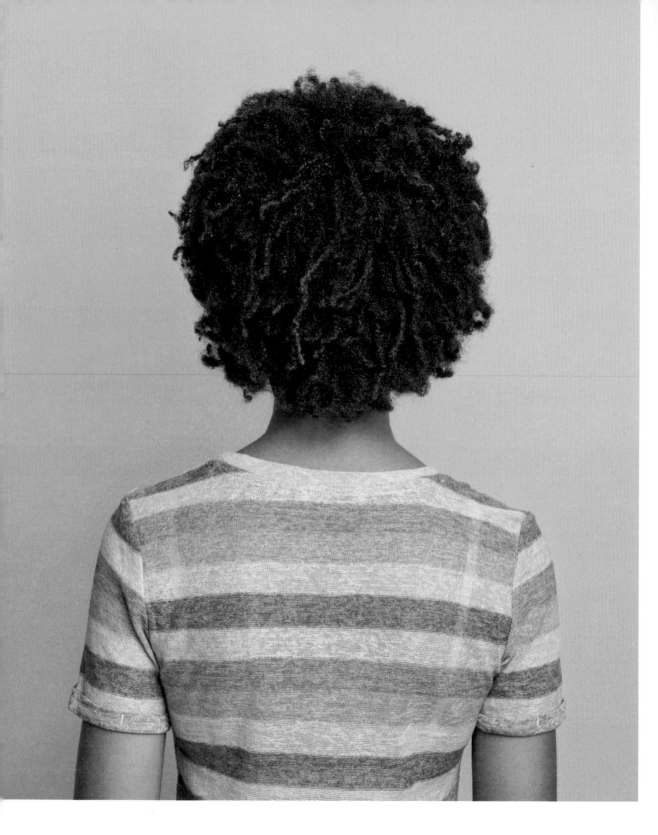

Keep Your Mane Healthy + Strong

A good self-care haircare routine doesn't need to be complicated. You need to focus on two things: keep your scalp healthy and protect your hair. To accomplish this, you only need to add an additional ninety seconds to your standard shampoo and conditioning routine.

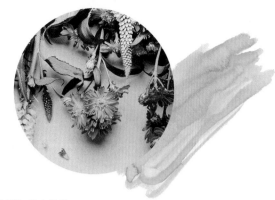

SCALP CARE

Keeping your scalp healthy will help your hair grow, minimize dry, flaky skin, keep oil production in check, help stop hair breakage, and decrease scalp irritation.

Try to limit washing your hair to two to three times a week to allow the production of the natural oils that keep your scalp healthy. Once a week, add an exfoliating step to stimulate your scalp, remove buildup, and let new hair grow in a healthy environment.

You can exfoliate your scalp two different ways.

① **Use a silicone scalp-massaging shampoo brush.** You can buy this online or in a beauty store. They're inexpensive and make your standard shampoo and conditioner routine more luxurious and effective. Simply shampoo your hair as you normally would, but use the brush, which hooks between your fingers, to scrub the shampoo into your scalp instead of using your fingers. The brush is easy to use, and it helps remedy scalp buildup.

② **Use a simple at-home exfoliating scrub.** Combine one part raw cane sugar with three parts conditioner and a few drops of tea tree oil. Wet your hair with warm water and scrub the mixture into your scalp using your fingers to give yourself a soothing massage. Rinse out thoroughly and then shampoo and condition as per your usual routine.

HAIR CARE

Invest in a good shampoo and conditioner that are made for your hair type. The combination that you use should be hypoallergenic and fragrance-free to avoid irritation. You might have to try out a few different shampoo and conditioner combinations until you find the one that you love, so have fun with the experience. It should be enjoyable because you are caring for yourself by giving your hair the products that it needs and deserves.

If you "heat style" your hair by blow drying, straightening, or curling it, you should take extra care to add hydration back into your strands. Simply add argan oil to your post-heat routine. Argan oil is a lightweight oil that will not compromise your hair's volume. It has a host of benefits, including:[13]

- Very moisturizing
- Promotes hair growth
- Seals split ends
- Fights frizz
- Produces shine

To apply to your locks, put two to three drops of argan oil in your hands, rub your palms together, and smooth the oil over the ends of your hair. Avoid the scalp because it naturally produces its own oils.

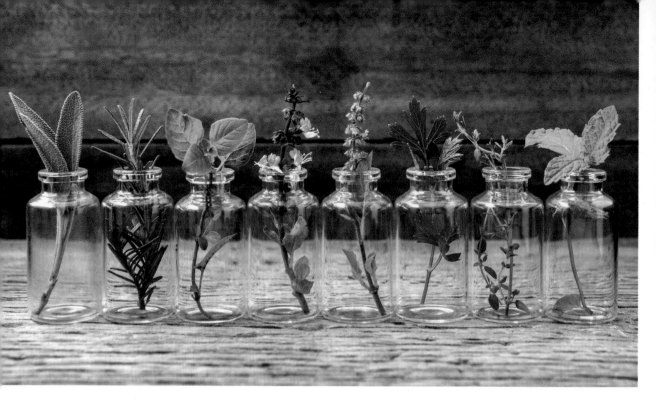

How Oils Can Benefit Your Beauty, Body, + Mind

Essential oils are a self-care must. You can use essential oils in many ways; aromatherapy, massage oil, scented bath oil, skin moisturizer, perfume, hair conditioner, or cuticle treatment. You can also use essential oils to scent a room.

Here's a quick guide to a few incredible oils and suggestions on how you can include them in your beauty routine and your life:

Lavender Oil:[14] This is the first oil you should incorporate into your oil arsenal if you're new to the world of essential oils. It helps with a host of mental struggles such as anxiety and can assist with sleep, helping you fall asleep faster and stay asleep longer. Try sprinkling some lavender oil onto your pillow for an extra-sound sleep. Using a mixture of castile soap and lavender oil can get rid of bacteria on your makeup brushes.

Tea Tree Oil:[15] This oil is very strong and should be diluted with a carrier oil before you put it on your skin. Use one part tea tree oil to ten parts carrier oil, such as almond oil or coconut oil. This mixture can help balance your skin, prevent dryness, soothe your scalp, and fight acne. You can use this mixture of tea tree oil and carrier oil on your skin or as a deep scalp treatment (wash well after leaving it on for 10-30 minutes).

Jojoba Oil:[16] Safe for all skin types, this oil penetrates deeply into your skin. You can use jojoba oil in your skincare routine for serious hydration or as a makeup remover and on your hair before washing it for a deep conditioning treatment. If your nails need some TLC, use jojoba oil to moisturize dry cuticles and nail beds.

Goddess Bath

A Goddess Bath is exactly what it sounds like—a bath fit for a goddess. You deserve to feel pampered, and this luxurious beauty ritual is a great way to show yourself love and self-care. You can save this bath for a special occasion or treat yourself to this relaxing ritual whenever you need to relax and recharge.

To create a Goddess Bath, you can use:

- Essential oils
- Non-toxic candles
- Soothing music
- Flowers and flower petals
- Crystals
- Aromatherapy bubble bath
- Bath bomb
- Hot oil hair treatment
- Face mask
- Homemade bath soaking salts

Imagine yourself in a warm bathtub full of flower petals with candles and crystals all around you. Your tension instantly melts away as you listen to soothing music and inhale your favorite scent. Now that's a Goddess Bath!

Make this dream a reality. You can start by making this easy, two-ingredient, homemade bath soaking salt.

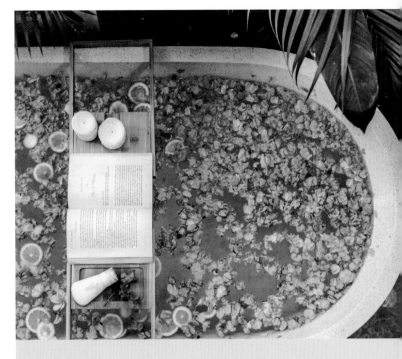

RECIPE

Goddess Bath Soaking Salts

You'll need:

Glass jar with a lid

Ingredients:

Epsom salt

Jasmine oil

① Fill the glass jar with Epsom salt. Put at least thirty drops of jasmine oil (feel free to add more) on the salts. Put the lid on the jar and shake well to incorporate the oils.

② While filling a bath with very warm water, place two heaping scoops of the scented bath salts under the running water. Swirl the water with your hands to dissolve the salts. Besides smelling delicious, scented bath salts help soothe aching muscles and remove impurities.

Sleep

Do you get enough sleep? Most of us do not. Adults need between seven and nine hours of sleep a night.[17] If you think that you don't have enough hours in the day to get this amount of sleep, the following sleep benefits might encourage you to prioritize sleep as an act of necessary self-care.

The Benefits of Sleep

Feeling well-rested is one obvious benefit of getting a good night's sleep. These other not-so-obvious benefits should be the motivation you need to get more shuteye:[18]

———

- Reduces stress and your risk of depression
- Improves your memory and makes you more alert
- Gives your body time to heal and repair itself
- Can help you lose weight
- Assists with heart health and preventing cancer

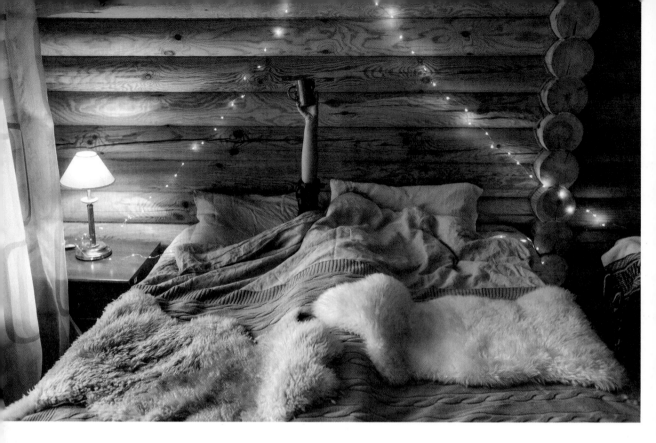

Light Cycles + Your Circadian Rhythm

Exposure to the correct amount of sunlight and darkness at the correct times of day or night can have a significant impact on how you function. Sunlight tells specific areas of your eye's retina to trigger your brain to release serotonin, a hormone known to battle depression and lift your mood. Darkness tells your brain to release melatonin, the hormone that helps you sleep.[19] When timed correctly, the right amount of light and darkness can increase joy and improve the quality of your sleep. Being happy and well-rested are self-care priorities.

The presence of light and dark assist in setting your *circadian rhythm*.[20] This is your 24-hour internal clock that affects the physical, behavioral, and mental elements of daily life. Daylight cues your circadian rhythm's timing. Not only does your circadian rhythm regulate sleep, but it also influences and regulates your hormones, body temperature, bodily functions, eating habits, and digestion. If you think of yourself as a car, daylight is the gasoline you need to make sure your vehicle is running properly.

Bye Bye, Blue Light

Blue light, or the light used in electronic screens and certain energy-efficient lighting, can disrupt sleep if you're exposed to it a few hours before bedtime.[21] This is because blue light disrupts the production of the hormone melatonin. Without enough melatonin, you won't have sufficient rest.

You can help lessen the effects of blue light by shutting down all electronic devices—smartphones, iPads, laptops—a few hours before bed, wearing blue-light blocking glasses, or eliminating screen time from your evening routine entirely.

Light Cycling Sleep Training Exercise

To set your circadian rhythm, you can use light and the absence of light to train your body. This can also improve mood stability and sleep issues in only a week.

To further enhance this exercise, you can create your ideal sleep sanctuary: control the temperature in your room and incorporate the use of soothing essential oils (covered in the next section).

STEP ONE: For seven days in a row (at a minimum, you can do more), set your alarm clock to wake you at the exact same time every day, including the weekends.

STEP TWO: Upon waking, immediately head outside and find the sun. Sit comfortably with your face turned toward the sun, eyes open (but not directly staring into the sun), and your palms facing upward. Slowly breathe in this position for ten minutes to mindfully start your day while you absorb sunlight and signal to your brain that it's daytime. It's time to begin your day and time for your brain to release serotonin to increase your happiness and energy.

STEP THREE: Maintain the same bedtime for seven days in a row (at a minimum, you can do more). Set an alarm to go off three hours before your bedtime as a reminder that you'll need to shut off all sources of blue light.

STEP FOUR: Turn off all screens and make sure you dim the lights in your home or use low-wattage light in the evenings. If you can't avoid screens entirely, use blue-light blocking glasses or download an app on your phone that blocks blue light.

STEP FIVE: You should notice that you sleep more soundly and wake up with renewed emotional stability, focus, and energy after a week of resetting your circadian rhythm.

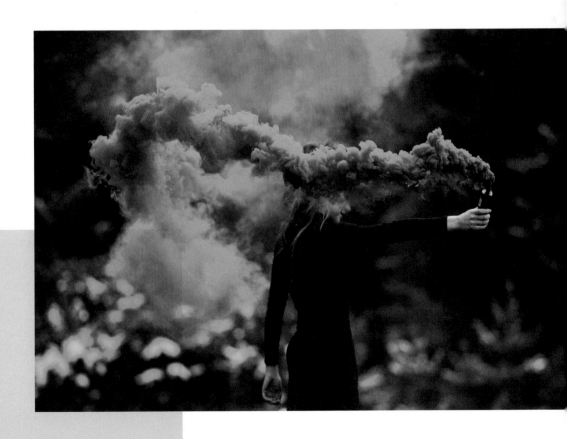

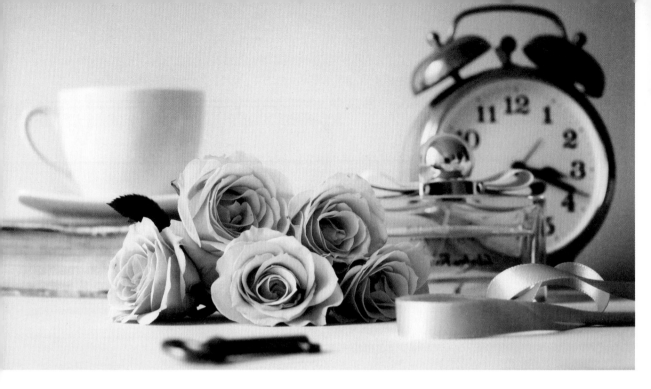

SLEEPING TIPS

There are ways you can improve your sleep and create the ideal conditions for a great night of refreshing rest.[22]

- **Temperature:** The ideal sleeping temperature is between 60°F and 67°F. Make sure your environment meets these conditions.

- **Light:** Any external source of light can interrupt your natural sleep cycle. Block all sources of external light from entering your bedroom while you're sleeping.

- **Sound:** Sleeping next to someone who snores or a noisy neighborhood can disrupt your sleep. Find a way to restrict this noise (earplugs are always an option).

- **Physical Activity:** A body that has moved during the day is a body that's more capable of resting during the night.

- **Sleep Schedule:** Get up at the same time each day and go to sleep at the same time each night (including weekends!). This helps your body's internal clock, which in turn helps you get a more restful sleep.

- **Pillows and Bedding:** Replace your mattress every ten years for ideal support. Use cozy, allergen-free pillows and bedding.

- **Essential Oils:** Soothing oils like lavender and bergamot signal the brain to relax.

- **Bedroom Sanctuary:** The bedroom is for sleeping (and sex!). Remove all screens from your bedroom and don't do your work on your bed. You want to associate your bedroom with relaxation.

- **Relaxation:** Creating an evening ritual reminds your body that it's time to slow down, relax, and prepare for rest.

- **Caffeine, Alcohol, and Food (Especially Sugar):** When you are preparing yourself for bed, avoid all of these substances because they can interfere with a peaceful night of rest.

Creating Your Sleep Sanctuary

This step-by-step exercise consolidates the tips above into an actionable plan. Set aside a few hours to consciously shop, choose the items that will create a cozy and comfortable environment, and then set up your space to set the foundation for a more peaceful slumber. Here's what you can do:

1. Invest in quality bedding that feels good against your skin. Buy pillows that support and cradle your neck and head and a mattress or mattress topper that protects your back.

2. Get a fan or use air conditioning to keep your room cool.

3. Buy blackout curtains and hang them on every window.

4. Remove all screens and work-related items from your room.

5. Get an air filter, humidifier, or white noise machine to block out disruptive sounds.

6. Keep a lavender scented candle and/or lavender oil in your room and use it nightly.

7. Invest in a dimmer for the light in your room or dimmable side table lamps to create a peaceful and relaxing environment before bed.

8. Get ready for the sleep you deserve.

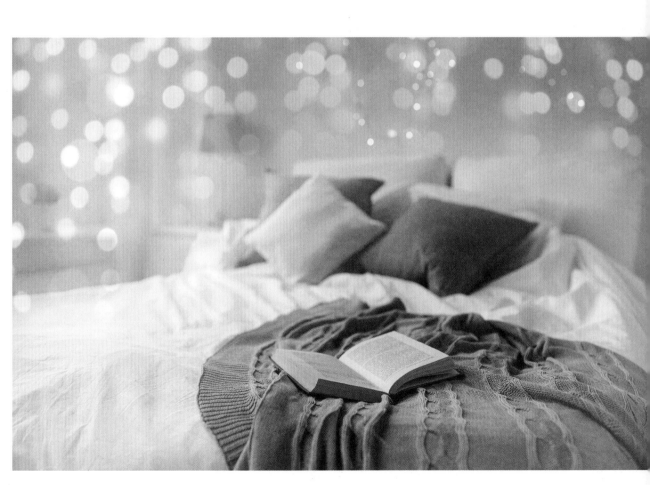

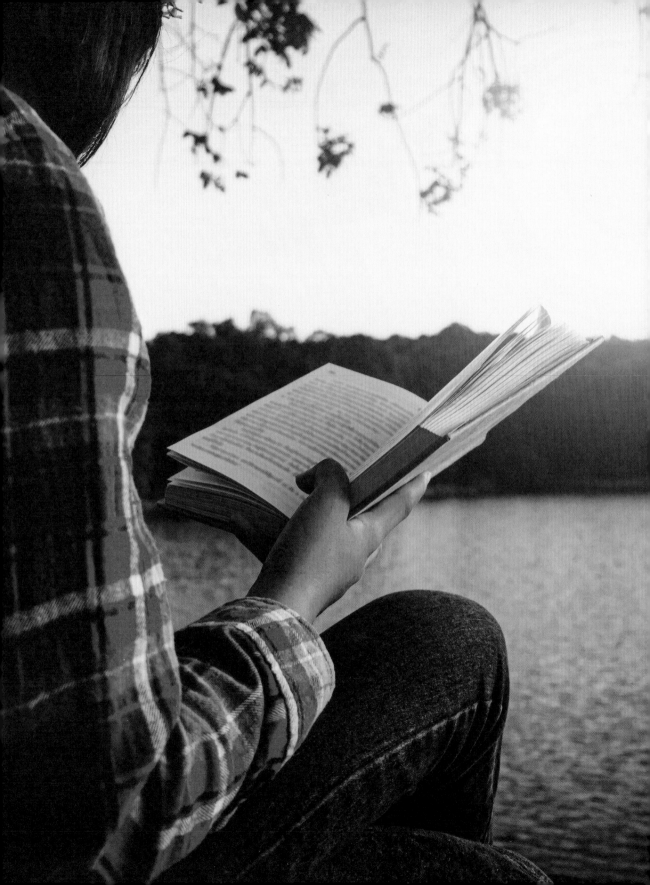

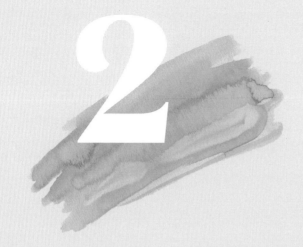

INTELLECTUAL
SELF-CARE

*"Imagination
is more important
than knowledge."*

—ALBERT EINSTEIN

Create

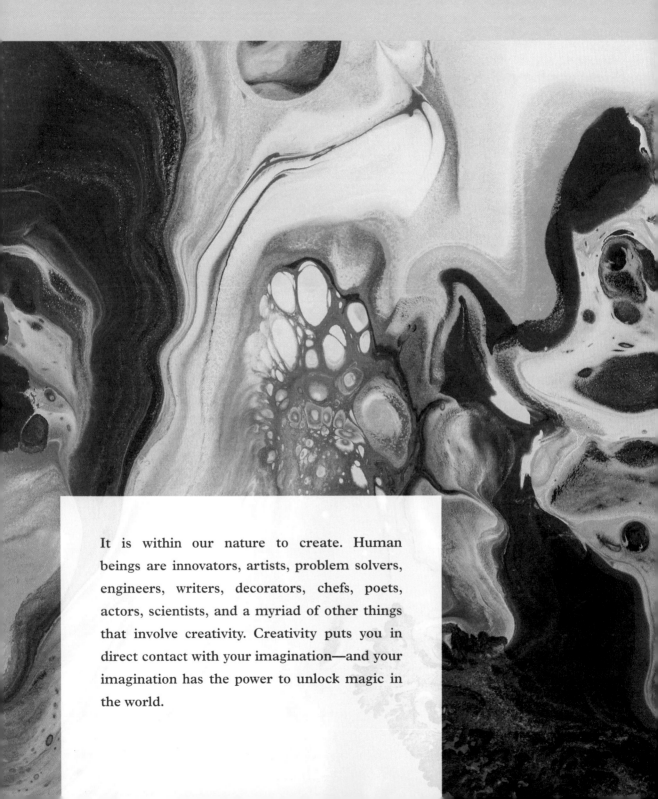

It is within our nature to create. Human beings are innovators, artists, problem solvers, engineers, writers, decorators, chefs, poets, actors, scientists, and a myriad of other things that involve creativity. Creativity puts you in direct contact with your imagination—and your imagination has the power to unlock magic in the world.

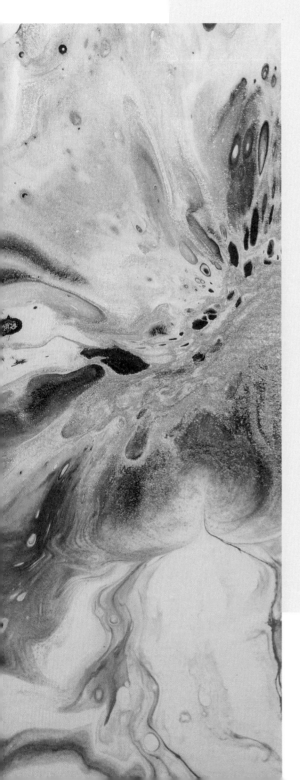

Everyone is an Artist

Being an artist has nothing to do with being "good" or "bad" at creating. Art is just that—art.

———

When you were a child, you likely found a great deal of joy in finger painting and whether the outcome was objectively beautiful or not, it didn't stop you from enjoying the process of creation. You also probably colored as a kid and found joy in it, even if the colors ended up outside of the lines.

To put you back in touch with the artist within, you must remove your attachment to the outcome. Don't worry about whether or not the final product will be worth framing—the true joy of being an artist is the process of creation, not the end result. Removing the need to be "good" at creating allows you to tap into the imaginative freedom you relied on as a child.

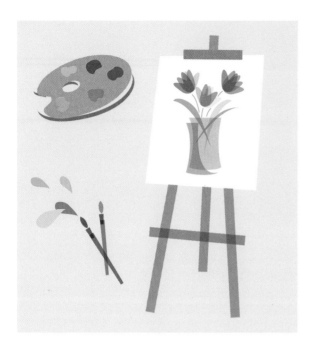

PAINTING 101

The first step is to simply begin. If you need a jumping off point to begin painting, start with these basics:

- **Get a few blank canvases.** You can find these online or at your local art or craft store.

- **Use acrylic paint in primary colors, black, and white.** This paint can also be found online or at your local art or craft store. Acrylic paints are a good paint to start with because they mix easily, have a smooth consistency, and dry relatively quickly. You can mix red, yellow, and blue paint to create other colors. Incorporating white will lighten the colors and using black on the canvas can create depth, lines, and shadow.

- **Get cardboard or an artist's palette.** You can mix colors and create a variety of shades on this.

- **Find some good paintbrushes.** You only need two brushes to begin: a round brush and a pointed round brush. More advanced brushes can be obtained later.

- **Set up your easel.** This is optional because you may have a preference as to whether you want to use an easel when you paint.

- **Fill a cup with water.** You use water to rinse your brushes after use or when switching between colors.

Once you're ready to begin painting, find objects, ideas, colors, and images that really inspire you.

There is so much beauty in the world, and you are the channel that transmits those joys into art. If you are not quite sure where to start or what your first muse should be, you can:

① **Free Paint:** This type of painting asks you to ignore what you may end up creating and instead, is all about enjoying the process. Mix a variety of colors until you create shades you love. Paint on the canvas and layer the paint with reckless abandon—don't think about what the final product will be. Simply enjoy the process of creation and allow your creativity to flow. Think of this as your version of abstract art.

② **Landscape:** Imagine a simple and calming landscape. Maybe it's a field under a bright blue sky. Or a mountain range with a sunset. Perhaps you're envisioning a lone tree on a hillside. Imagine the vista in your mind and then try to get the colors to match the colors in your imagination. Take your time mixing your shades and start by painting simple lines. Enjoy watching your vision come to life.

③ **Vase of Flowers:** The best part of this exercise is that the first step is going out and buying yourself flowers! Next, arrange them in a vase and sit back and observe. Try to match the shape of the vase and the colors of the flowers. Notice how your eyes see the vase, your mind translates the colors and the shapes, your imagination begins to add its own spin, and your hand brings your vision to life with brushstrokes on a canvas.

Vision Board:
What it is + How to Use it

A vision board is a visual representation of the dreams, hopes, and goals you have for your life. It's a powerful tool that helps you visualize the life you desire and helps you focus your mind on positivity to help facilitate your desires.

A vision board is helpful because it is a source of visual motivation. Because of this, you should put your vision board in a spot you look at every day. On days when you're feeling lost, confused about the direction of your life, or stuck in a rut, you can look at your vision board for a boost of optimism and a reminder of what you want out of life. On days when you're feeling happy, confident, and inspired, you can look at your vision board for ideas on how to channel your positive energy to get one step closer to your dream life.

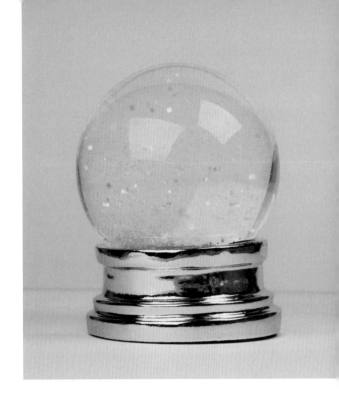

Creating A Vision Board

Creating a vision board is a fun pastime that utilizes your creativity and helps serve as a reminder of the life you're working to manifest. It serves your self-care routine in the following ways: it allows you to tap into your childlike creativity and sense of play, and it also serves as a motivational tool.

You'll need:

Music that makes you feel inspired

A bulletin board or poster board

Scissors

Numerous magazines

Push pins (if using a bulletin board) or a glue stick (if using a poster board)

(1) Set out all of your materials on a large work surface.

(2) Play inspiring music and sit for five minutes with your eyes closed. During this time, imagine—in vivid detail—the things that would bring you the most joy. Imagine your day-to-day routine, your career, your love life, your social life, your wardrobe—everything down to the smallest details like your favorite breakfast.

(3) Open your eyes and begin flipping through the magazines. Cut out photos and words that fit the vision you imagined. If you lose focus, close your eyes and visualize again for another five minutes or step away from the exercise for an hour and then come back to it.

(4) Once you've cut out several images and words, attach them to the bulletin board or poster board with the push pins or the glue, respectively.

(5) Once you've attached the images and words to the board, locate a place to hang it. Make sure to display it in a room or spot you're in every day.

(6) Look at your vision board each morning to set your intention for the day as a reminder that you have many things to work toward and feel hopeful about. Your vision board is the key to creating the life you deserve.

Music

Music has the power to evoke memory, capture a moment, and shift a mood. It's a powerful form of self-care because it directly impacts your brain immediately. When you hear music you enjoy, your brain releases dopamine, a chemical that positively shifts your mood by rewarding your brain.[23] Music provides a host of additional benefits:

- Lessens stress and decreases anxiety
- Improves memory and cognitive function
- Eases physical and emotional pain
- Increases feelings of comfort and connection

You can bring music into your life by attending a live show, making your own music, or curating a playlist of music that brings you joy.

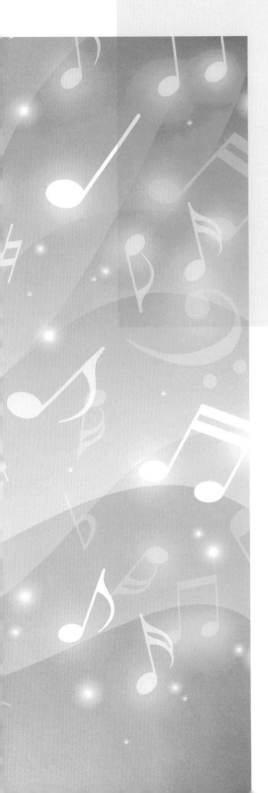

Simple Instruments

You don't have to be musically inclined to create your own music. Start with one of the following simple instruments and allow yourself to learn—and play—at your own pace.[24] This is about enjoying the experience of connecting with the instrument and figuring out what kind of music you like.

Ukulele: Whereas a guitar has six strings and can take a bit longer to master, the ukulele has only four strings, which cuts down on the amount of time it takes to learn chords and play simple songs. The ukulele is a relatively affordable and small instrument that won't take up a lot of space in your home.

Bongos: This simple instrument is comprised of two wrapped drums that are connected. To play it, hit your hand on top of the instrument. You can experiment with creating different drum beats by hitting the tops of the drums in different locations, with different parts of your hand and palm, and with different levels of force and rhythm.

Glockenspiel: This small instrument looks like a miniature xylophone; it has tiny metal bars you hit with sticks for a happy, tinny sound. This is a great instrument to have in your home because you can easily store it in a drawer or on a shelf, and start playing it without any formal training.

Harmonica: This inexpensive instrument is portable, and you can begin playing it right away. Start by blowing with different levels of force and sliding the harmonica from side to side to find the different notes you can create. Then start to use your hand to cover the harmonica and control the air flow out of the instrument for even more rhythmic control.

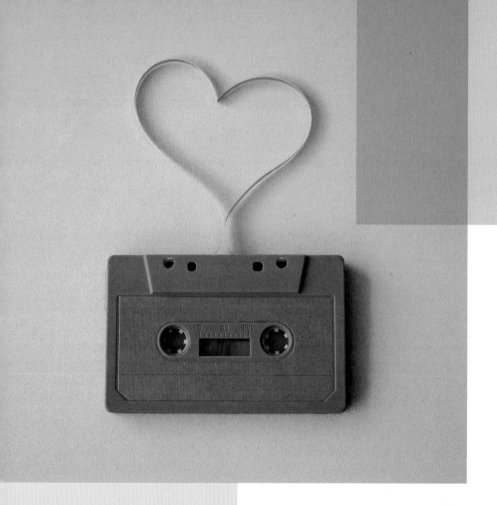

The Happy Playlist

A happy playlist is exactly what it sounds like: a music playlist that makes you happy. Taking the time to create and curate this playlist is a beautiful exercise in self-care.

You can cue up your happy playlist anywhere and at any time. Play it in the car, at home, in your headphones on a walk, or connect it to a speaker and share your playlist with a group of friends. Listen to it when you're happy to make yourself even happier. Play it when you're feeling stuck or sad to remind your brain of the happier times and to put you in a better mood. This playlist will be ready and waiting for you when you feel like you need a boost.

Here's how to create your happy playlist

STEP ONE: Brainstorm. Sit down with a piece of paper and a pen and think about the songs that make you happy. These should be songs that instantly lift your mood, that you connect with, and that make you want to sing and dance. Write them down.

STEP TWO: Go through your music collection. Since music is now primarily digital, scroll through your phone's music library, the music stored on your computer, and any music you have saved on a digital music platform (like Spotify, Pandora, or Apple Music). Find the songs that make you happy and add them to the list you started making in Step One.

STEP THREE: Take note of the music you choose to listen to when you're happy or feeling good. This could be the radio station that you turn on in the car or the songs you find yourself playing that feel like "anthems" to you. Add these to your list.

STEP FOUR: Create a digital playlist from your list of songs. Use your music service provider (if you don't have one, Spotify and Apple Music are both simple to use and have large music libraries) to locate the songs on your list. Add them to a playlist titled "Happy."

STEP FIVE: Rearrange the order of the songs on your playlist until the flow makes sense to you. Now you have the ultimate happy soundtrack for your life!

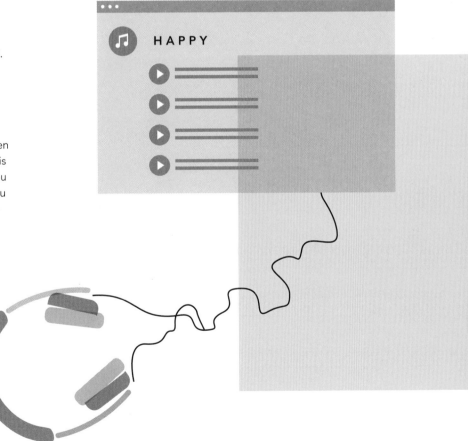

HAPPY

Writing

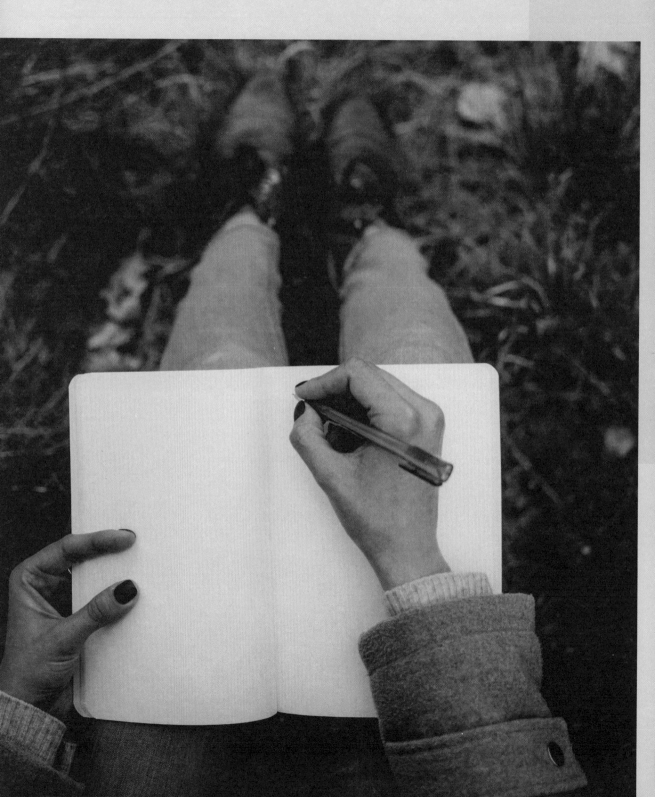

The written word is so important. Writing is how we can communicate with each other and it's also a way you can communicate with yourself, tapping into your thoughts, identifying and releasing yourself from your fears, and manifesting your dreams. When you take time to put your thoughts on paper, you're providing space to understand yourself more fully so that you can live a more authentic life.

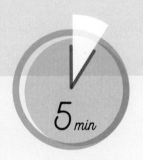

Morning Pages: How Five Minutes Can Reduce Anxiety

Setting aside five minutes each morning to connect with yourself is one of the most important things you can do to set yourself up for a good day. If you don't have five minutes in the morning to write, set your alarm five minutes earlier than normal. These extra five minutes can have a massive impact on the rest of your day if you use them correctly.

If you make it a daily habit, the following exercise can reduce anxiety, increase joy, and help you focus. How does it work? Your morning pages let you acknowledge and let go of pain points. It gives you clear, achievable objectives for the day, helps set your mood, and shifts you to a space of gratitude, imagination, and hope. This exercise is so effective it can feel like you took a magic mood-boosting pill.

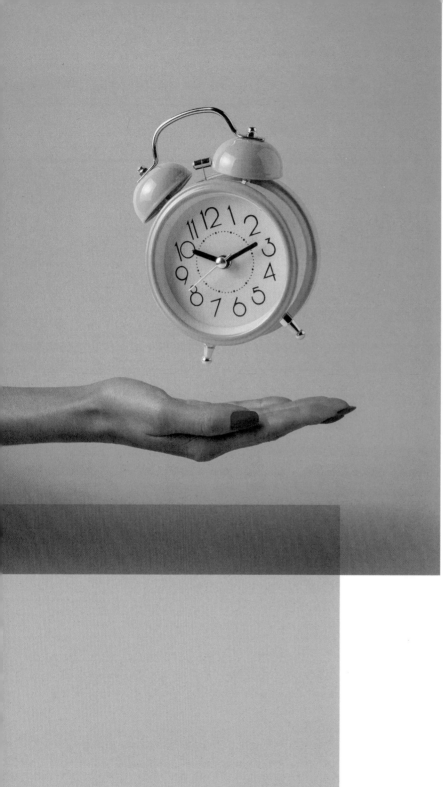

Your Morning Pages

You'll need:

A pen you love to write with

A blank piece of white paper

(1) Write the day of the week and the date at the top of the paper as a title (example: Friday, July 13, 2023).

(2) Write the following sections on your paper with space in between each section: Thoughts, To Be Completed, Intention, Gratitude, and Dreams. Put these sections anywhere you want on the page. The flow of the page is up to you.

(3) Under the heading To Be Completed, make six check boxes with spaces next to them for room to write.

(4) Under the headings Gratitude and Dreams, write the numbers one through three in a list form.

(5) Get creative with how your page looks, but it might look something like this. →

Friday.
July 13. 2023

Thoughts:

To be completed:

- ☐ _____
- ☐ _____
- ☐ _____

- ☐ _____
- ☐ _____
- ☐ _____

Intention:

Gratitude:

1.

2.

3.

Dreams:

1.

2.

3.

(6) Now that your paper is ready for you, it's time to fill in each section:

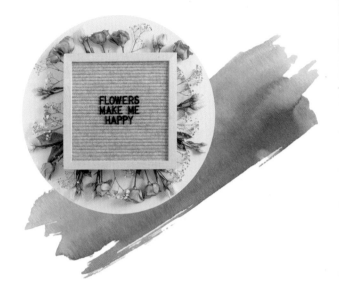

- **Thoughts:** Write freely. You may find that you wake up and have anxious thoughts about the day ahead or maybe you feel tired. Maybe you're excited or perhaps you feel a little foggy. Write it out. Honestly, these words don't even need to make sense. Put anything and everything you're thinking about in this section. Get it out of your head and on to the page. This helps you clear space for the thoughts that you want to consciously put into your mind.

- **To Be Completed:** Jot down no more than six goals for the day. They can be big or small. They can feel significant or trivial. But they should all be achievable within a single day. You can write anything from "eat a balanced breakfast" to "crush the work presentation" to "spend thirty minutes in a bubble bath." Use this section to get a clear view of your objectives for the day and—this is important—celebrate each time you check something off the list. You can give yourself a standing ovation, dance around the room, or do a quick fist pump. By celebrating your victories—big and small—you train your mind to act like your biggest cheerleader.

- **Intention:** Write down who you want to show up as today. It can say something like "I am patient and loving and an active listener," or "I am a bright white light," or "I am powerful and confident and will help lead others by example."

Whatever you write here should reflect the best version of yourself. When you write it down, you form a mental commitment to your intention. You can then draw on your intention throughout the day to bring yourself back to center and stay focused on who you want to be.

- **Gratitude:** Write down three very specific things you're grateful for. Nothing is too big or too small because the simple act of gratitude gives even the little things weight. You can write something like "my best friend who will pick up my phone call at 3 a.m.," or "the sturdy roof over my head," or "the bright toenail polish I'm wearing," or "sunshine, clean water, and freedom." Again, whatever you write here just has to be true to you. Bonus points if you read your gratitude list out loud after writing it.

- **Dreams:** This is another area where you need to be very specific. Write *exactly* what you're hoping for, wishing for, or manifesting for your future. You can write the specifics of your dream bedroom. Or your dream man. Your dream job. You can dream of world peace. Or equality. Whatever it is, dream it, write it, and watch it come true.

(7) Put this list up in a place where you'll see it often throughout the day. It can go in your planner or snap a photo of it and make it your phone backdrop. You can hang it on the fridge or put it up on a bulletin board. You want to put this sheet of paper in a convenient place so that in the midst of the day's hustle and bustle, you can look at it and remember how grateful, clear, and calm you were when you wrote it.

(8) Repeat this exercise daily to live a happier, more effective, and purposeful life.

Gratitude Journal

One of the best things you can do for your mindset is to adopt an *attitude of gratitude*. Learning to be grateful for the smallest things is one of the quickest ways to have a happy life. Sometimes it can be hard to see the good things in your life, especially when overwhelm, exhaustion, or emotional pain enter the picture.

In these moments of pain, it's especially important to have a list of things you're grateful for. You can reread them as a reminder of all of the good that does exists—even when the bad clouds your ability to see it.

Starting a gratitude journal is an amazing way to guarantee that you'll always have something to read—a book of your own creation—that can lift your spirits.

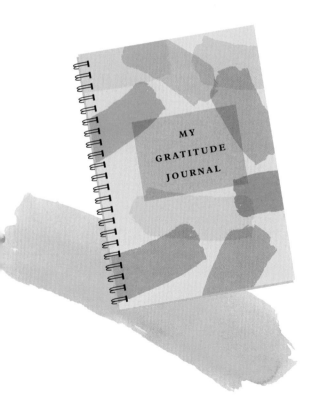

Gratitude Journal

You'll need:

A spiral-bound, lined notebook

A pen you love to write with

(1) Keep the journal next to your bed.

(2) Before you go to sleep, open the journal and starting on the first page on the top line, begin your list by writing a "1." Then follow the number with something you're grateful for.

(3) Continue numbering and adding gratitude items each night (example: on the second night, you'll write "2" on the empty line below your first entry. Write down something you're grateful for after the number two.

(4) Continue this practice for as long as you're alive! Refer to this list in your journal any time you feel pain as a reminder of the beautiful things you already have in your life.

(5) At the end of a year, you'll have a book of 365 things for which you're unbelievably grateful.

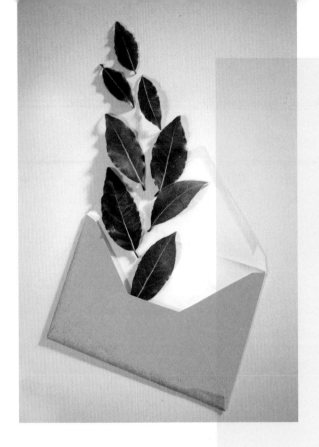

Writing Letters to Yourself

Living in the past—where regret, second-guessing, loss, grief, and painful memories exist—can cause you to feel depressed. Living in the future—where fear, confusion, control issues, unknowns, and a series of "what-ifs" exist—can cause you to feel anxious. Getting you to a place where you can embrace the present moment will increase your awareness, gratitude, and self-love, which are all components of self-care. The following exercises involve writing letters to yourself as a way to clear your internal blocks and make way for love.

Letter to Your Past Self

You'll need:

A pen you love to write with

Blank sheets of white paper

A lighter or matches

A fire-safe place for disposal
(a fire pit, a non-flammable
bin/bucket, etc.)

Sit down in a calm, quiet location. Close your eyes and breathe in and out slowly for one minute to center yourself. Then write yourself a letter addressing things that have happened in the past. This may take you a while to write. Be patient and gentle with yourself during this process. You can write down things from the past that have hurt you or loss you've experienced. Write about things you need to forgive yourself for or advice your current self would give your younger self. There are no rules for what you can write about—the only requisite is that you write about things that happened in the past.

It's normal if you find this writing exercise emotionally exhausting. Sometimes self-care involves the acknowledgment of painful moments to help you fully release them.

After you have finished writing your letter, go someplace where you can light a fire safely. Close your eyes and internally acknowledge that you're ready to close the door on things from your past that are holding you back. Say good-bye to unhealthy patterns or lingering negativity from the past. Now light the letter on fire and as the words turn to ash, tell yourself that the pain inside of you is also disintegrating. Discard the burned letter in a fire-safe place of disposal.

Letter to Your Future Self

You'll need:

A pen you love to write with

A thick black marker

Blank sheets of white paper

A glass bottle with a lid/cork

A shovel

Without any external distractions, use the thin black marker to write a letter about your hopes, dreams, and even your fears. The only rule here is that everything you write about needs to be hypothetical and in the future—there should be nothing in this letter that has already come to fruition. Write candidly and openly. Allow yourself to explore your dreams and fears freely.

When you're done writing, take the thick black marker and cross off any fears you wrote down: this sends a signal to your mind that these fears are gone. Now you're only going to put thought and intention toward achieving your dreams. Roll up the letter and place it in a bottle. Find a location where you can dig a hole to bury it. Tell yourself that you're permanently burying your fears and planting a seed for your dreams to grow.

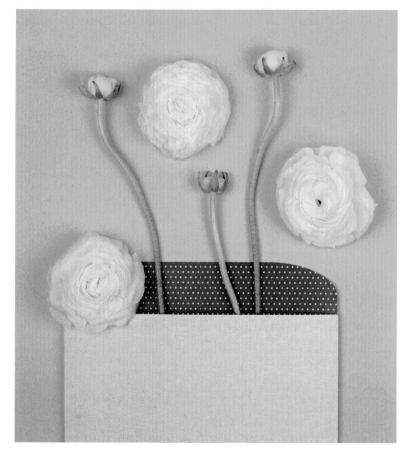

EXERCISE

Love Letter to Yourself

You'll need:

A pen you love to write with

Blank sheet of white paper

A picture frame that fits the sheet of paper

Write yourself a madly passionate love letter. Praise yourself. Pretend that you're the one true love of your life (spoiler: *you should be*). Focus on things that make you beautiful (physically, mentally, and emotionally), your unique qualities, your remarkable traits, or things you just really like/love about yourself. When you're done writing, frame your love letter and place it in a special spot. Read it every day until your loving thoughts about yourself become who you truly are.

Journal Prompts

On those days when you just cannot seem to get out of your own way–open a notebook, grab a pen, and respond to one of these journal prompts to get your creative juices flowing and to unblock yourself.

These prompts are effective because they shift your mind to a place of imagination and hope and force you to employ gratitude and optimism. The prompts also put you in a place where you must remove your self-limiting beliefs. The more you practice forcing your mindset to shift in this way the easier it will be to shift your mood on your own.

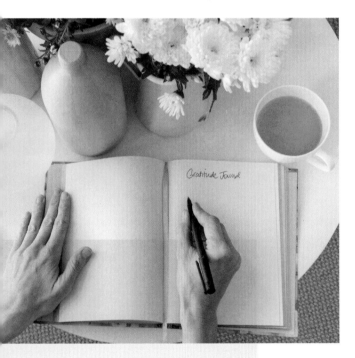

Here are ten prompts to get you out of a rut:

(1) What's your perfect day? Describe it in detail from morning to night.

(2) Write a tribute to your favorite person, and pretend it will be read aloud at an awards show held in his or her honor.

(3) A genie appears and grants you three wishes. What are they? Why did you wish for these things?

(4) You've just won $100 million and have seven days to spend it! Write the story of what happens during those seven days.

(5) A knock is at your door—it's a reality television show offering to build your dream house! They need to know where you want it built and what you want it to look like. What do you say?

(6) You have ten minutes to meet with the President of the United States. What you say in those ten minutes will greatly influence the President and the course of history. What do you say?

(7) You get to have dinner with anyone who has ever existed, living or dead. Who do you choose? What do you eat? What do you discuss?

(8) You have a time machine and can only use it once. What time period do you choose and why?

(9) You can go back as an adult to visit yourself as a child. What age do you revisit? Why? What advice or guidance do you give yourself, if any?

(10) You die at the age of one hundred. What does your obituary say?

Manifesting Goals

You'll need:

A scented candle you love

A spiral-bound notebook

A pen you love to write with

A blank piece of white paper

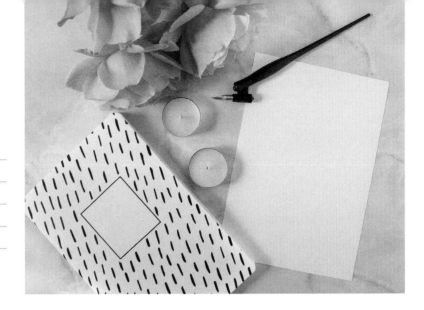

(1) Find a peaceful, comfortable, and quiet location. Light the candle and close your eyes. Breathe slowly and deeply—in through your nose and out through your mouth—for a few minutes until you reach a place of calm and focus.

(2) Imagine the following: each month, you'll get $500,000 directly deposited into your bank account, and you already have $100 million in the bank (so money is never an issue or an excuse to keep you from your dreams). You're ten years older, and you have complete freedom, no guilt, no obligations, no expectations from others. You're at a point in your life where you're blissfully happy.

(3) Open your spiral notebook. Write each and every detail—from your first moment of waking until you lay your head down to rest—of your day. For example:

- What time do you wake up?

- What does your bedroom look like?

- What's the first thing you do when you get up?

- Where do you live?

- Who do you live with?

- What do you eat for breakfast?

- How is your hair cut?

- How do you get ready?

Go through the minutia of your day. Each detail matters, and the clearer you can see it, the clearer you can write it. Clearly writing it means a clearer manifestation. The clearer you can manifest it, the faster you can begin living it.

(4) After you've finished writing every detail of a day in your life ten years from now—filled with pure happiness and zero limitations— imagine what *you are like at this stage in your life.*

(5) Write about yourself in detail. Use lots of adjectives. For example:

- Are you confident?

- Do you smile often?

- Are you helpful?

- Kind?

- Focused?

(6) Go back through this description of yourself and underline or circle the adjectives.

(7) On the blank piece of white paper, write down these adjectives.

(8) Take this piece of paper and tape it on your mirror. Read it every single morning and embody all of these qualities today.

(9) It's not your dream life that makes you into such an incredible person. It's being an incredible person that allows your dream life to become a reality.

(10) Start showing up as your *dream self today* and watch your dream life appear—in the form of increased joy—quickly.

Reading

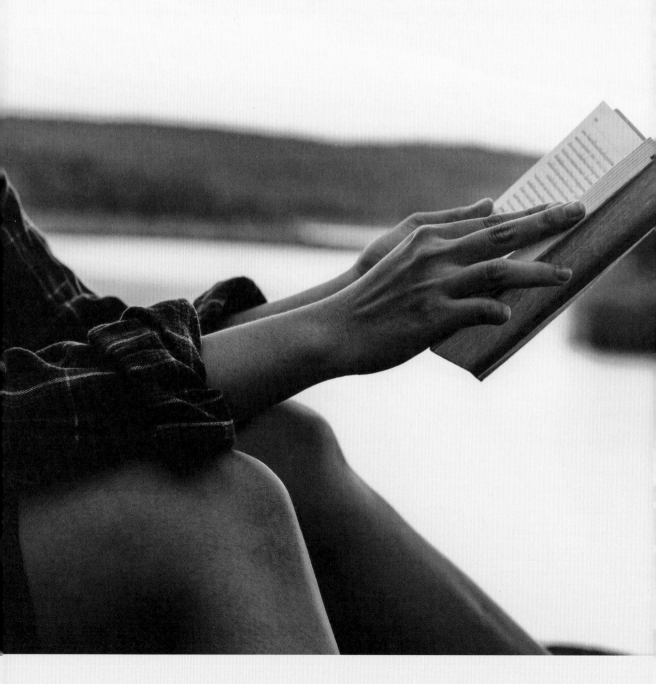

If you think of reading as a hobby, pastime, or optional activity, think again. Your brain needs a workout arguably more than your body. There are numerous worthwhile benefits to reading:[25]

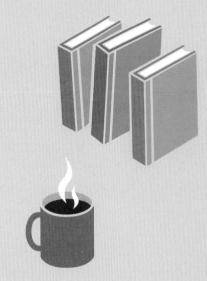

- Relieves stress
- Increases wisdom and knowledge
- Expands your vocabulary, which can help you express yourself and can increase self-confidence
- Improves your memory and helps fight dementia
- Improves your focus and concentration
- Provides entertainment and insight

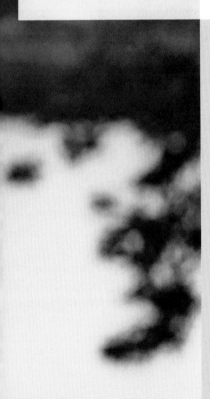

In your day to day existence, you are likely exposed to similar people, patterns, and experiences. When you read books written by someone else—whether they be fiction or non-fcition—you are instantly stepping into the mind, ideas, and perceptions of another entirely distinct individual. In this way, reading is one of the most efficient ways to expand your mind, broaden your worldview, and show your intellect some serious self-care. Taking 10 minutes a day to read something that someone else had written creates new connections in your mind and encourages neuroplasticity, which is your brain's ability to shift, change, and grow throughout your life. This daily brain workout can be heavy lifting—like a scientific article—or just a quick brain-walk-around-the-block with a simple beach read or magazine. Because this is self-care oriented, keep your focus on your enjoyment.

"Reading" With Your Ears

Technology is so advanced that you can now "read a book" by listening to it. There are a variety of apps and programs that let you download books and listen to them; you can pay for these apps or use the downloadable audio books provided for free by many local libraries.

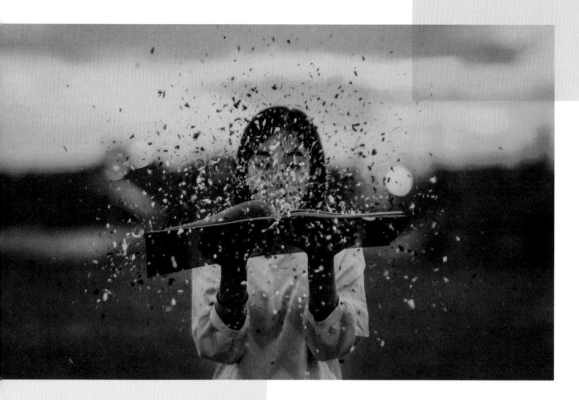

If you use this technology with intention, you can find time in your day to constantly "read" (by listening!) and learn. You can turn your car into a classroom by listening to a book on tape on your morning commute or while running errands. You can wear headphones or use a Bluetooth speaker to listen to an audio book while washing dishes, making dinner, stretching, folding laundry, or cleaning your house. You can go on a walk around your neighborhood and listen to an audio book to get your physical and mental exercise done at the same time.

Five Books to Add to Your Self-Care Arsenal

There are so many incredible print and audio books available. These five self-help and personal development books are a great jumping off point to help you further your self-care goals:

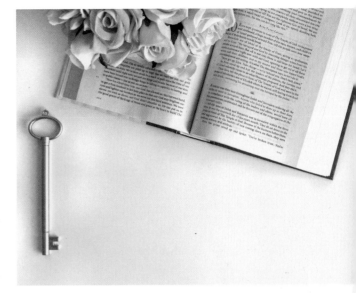

① *You are a Badass* by Jen Sincero: This book will leave you full of positivity and feeling like you can take on the world. It's like having a coach's halftime speech in your back pocket. Read it anytime you need a boost or a reminder that you already have everything you need to lead a happy and fulfilling life.

② *The Alchemist* by Paulo Coehlo: This must-read is a beautiful allegory about a shepherd boy who dreams of visiting the pyramids and, through a series of mystical encounters, goes on a magical journey against all odds. Different people interpret this book differently, and you'll see certain elements of yourself in the shepherd boy.

③ *Big Magic* by Elizabeth Gilbert: This book is a reminder that you're already a creative genius whether you know it or not. The author uses positive language and real-world examples to plug you back into your imagination and let your creative energy guide you.

④ *The Universe Has Your Back* by Gabrielle Bernstein: This book is like attending a weekend retreat that leaves you hopeful, refreshed, and convinced that everything in your life is happening for the highest good. Reading this book is a wonderful way to shift your mindset and learn more about the power of manifestation.

⑤ *The Four Agreements* by Don Miguel Ruiz: A classic self-help book, this quick read helps you remove mental obstacles and self-imposed blocks in your life. The strategies are highly beneficial and easy to apply.

Home

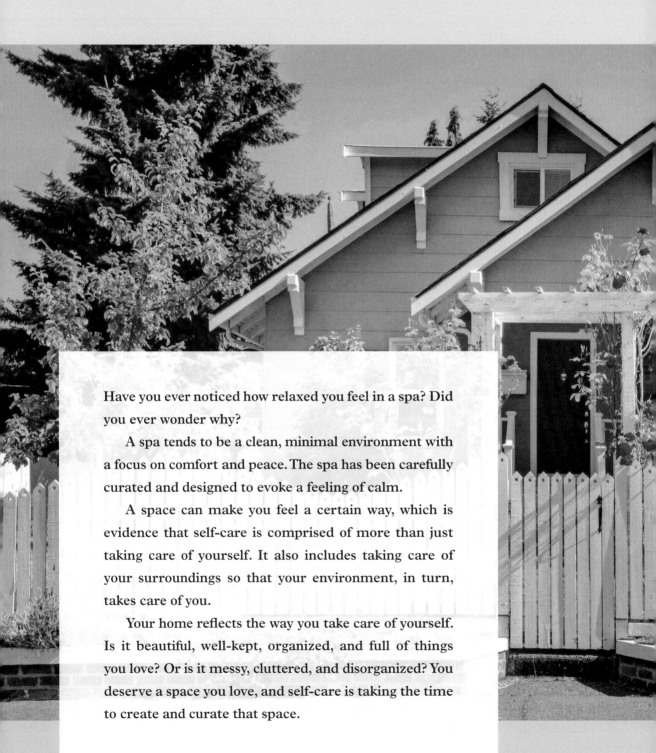

Have you ever noticed how relaxed you feel in a spa? Did you ever wonder why?

A spa tends to be a clean, minimal environment with a focus on comfort and peace. The spa has been carefully curated and designed to evoke a feeling of calm.

A space can make you feel a certain way, which is evidence that self-care is comprised of more than just taking care of yourself. It also includes taking care of your surroundings so that your environment, in turn, takes care of you.

Your home reflects the way you take care of yourself. Is it beautiful, well-kept, organized, and full of things you love? Or is it messy, cluttered, and disorganized? You deserve a space you love, and self-care is taking the time to create and curate that space.

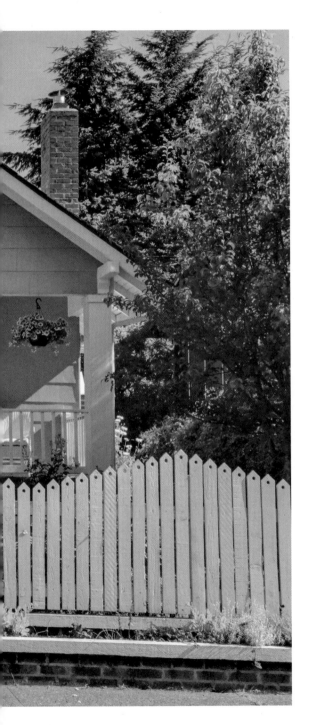

How Clutter Impacts Your Mindset

The world can be overwhelming enough without the added stress of coming home to a messy, disorganized, and cluttered space. You may not have control over the world, but you do have control over what's in your home.

———

There are many tangible psychological benefits to de-cluttering your space, including:[26]

- Making decisions about what stays and what goes increases your confidence, and you'll in turn see yourself as more competent.

- Organized spaces decrease anxiety and increase efficiency.

- De-cluttering your home is an energizing physical activity with tangible results: you can visibly see your progress. You know what you have (this keeps you from buying duplicates or having to search for an item, which wastes valuable time).

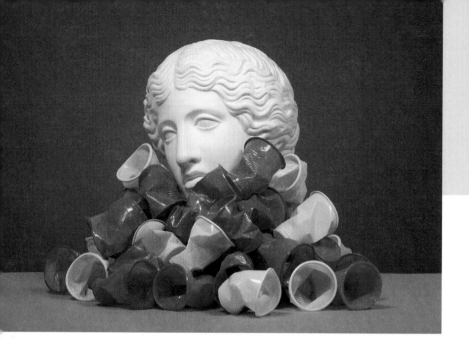

HOW TO KEEP
A CLUTTER-FREE HOME

Essentially, if an item isn't useful, isn't being used, or doesn't elicit a feeling of happiness, get rid of it. Go through this assessment for *every single item in your home*. Do this one room at a time (give yourself at least one full day for each room) until your space only includes items that assist you, either practically or emotionally.

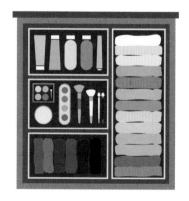

Here are seven things to donate or throw away:

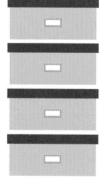

(1) Clothing that you haven't worn in the past year. Donate it if it's still in good condition.

(2) Financial paperwork that is more than seven years old. Shred it and put it in the recycling bin.

(3) Towels that are stained or have holes in them.

(4) Uncomfortable shoes, chairs, sheets, etc. If it's uncomfortable, it doesn't belong in your home.

(5) Anything that's expired in your fridge, pantry, or medicine cabinet.

(6) Any piece of a pair that's missing its other half. Example: a single sock or a single earring.

(7) Items that have gone unused for over a year.

Creating a Sanctuary

Think of the spa environment I mentioned earlier. You want to bring all of these elements into your space.

Here is a checklist to get your home a step closer to Zen:

- **Non-toxic Candles:** Buy them in scents that you love.
- **Pillows and Throws:** Incorporate comfortable pillows and throws to create a cozy atmosphere.
- **Dimmable Lighting:** This type of lighting lets you control the mood of a space.
- **Diffusers:** Use these with some of your favorite essential oils.
- **Robes and Slippers:** Wear these around the house so that you're comfortable in your sanctuary.

- **Temperature Control:** Use AC, fans, and heaters to keep your environment at the temperature of your liking.
- **Decorative Baskets:** Store clutter in large baskets in a centralized location. This way, you can go through the basket when you have time and return the item to its proper location.
- **Music:** If you don't have them already, invest in Bluetooth speakers so you can play mood-shifting music throughout your space.
- **Live Plants:** Real plants help to circulate fresh air in your home and add a natural element to your space.
- **Artwork:** Showcase works of art that evoke serenity and joy. Think of landscapes or a painting of the ocean.

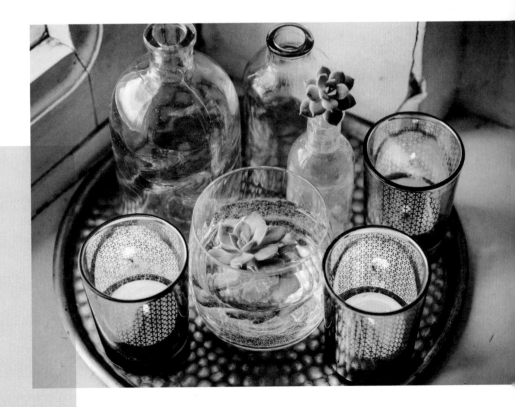

Remaining Childlike

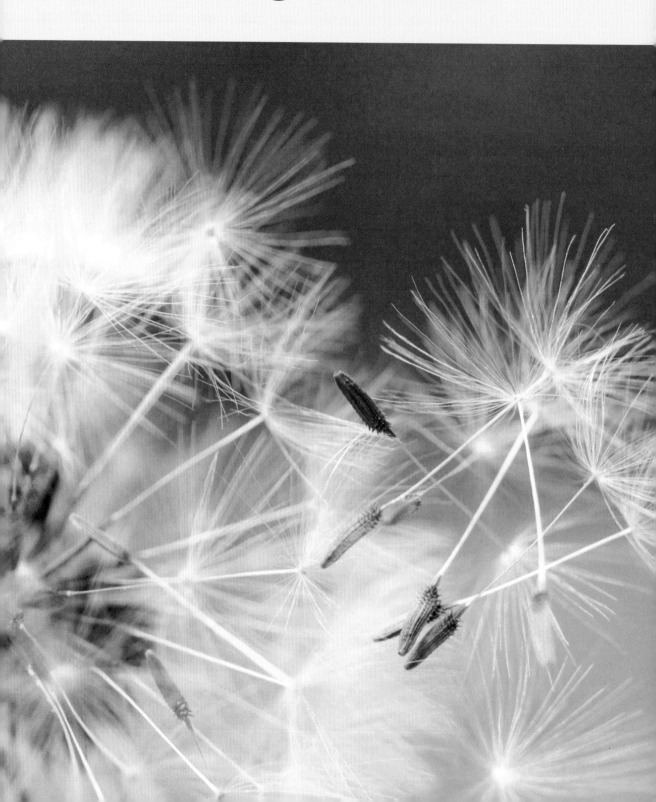

Many children inherently have a sense of wonder about the world. They can become fascinated with the littlest things and stay connected to the present moment. It's a child's fascinating connection to the world around him or her that makes childhood feel so magical. Through acts of self-care, you can reconnect with the magic of childhood and incorporate it into your adult identity.

This connection to your inner child can decrease anxiety, increase imagination and sense of self, unblock creativity, induce better sleep, and help infuse more joy into your life.

Awakening Your Inner Child

To connect with your inner child, you must plug back into the two components mentioned above:

———

① Fascination with simple things.

② Connection to the present moment and the world around you.

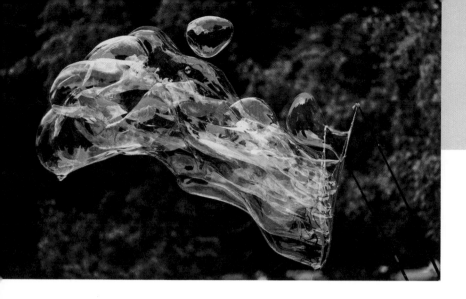

EXERCISES IN FASCINATION

Fascination can be reawakened by trying novel things without attachment to the outcome.

It can be difficult to remove outcome attachment because it is normal for your inner critic and perfectionist to show up and ruin the moment by telling you that whatever you're trying, doing, or creating "isn't good enough." The beautiful thing about being a child is that the outcome doesn't matter—it's the *doing* that provides joy.

But before you can become fascinated with something, you must remove "perfection" from your vocabulary. Your inner perfectionist and its chronic fear of failure will sabotage your chances at happiness.

Try incorporating the following activities into your life to silence the inner "perfectionist," a.k.a. your happiness saboteur:

Break something. Seriously. Take a stack of plates and go outside somewhere safe (wear protective clothing, footwear, and eyewear) and smash those plates! All of them. This is a strangely satisfying activity. When you were a child and you broke something, you didn't say, "Oh no!" until an adult taught you that you'd made a mistake. Before you learned to feel guilt, breaking things was fun because there was no attachment to the outcome. Remind your inner perfectionist that you like having a good time (and she's not invited to the party).

Go ahead and get messy. Run through the sprinklers barefoot and get mud on your feet. Eat a popsicle and let it drip down your chin. Bake brownies and lick the batter from the bowl. Put on your makeup using your fingers instead of a brush. The simple act of making a mess while having fun tells your inner perfectionist to quit being a killjoy.

Go outside and play. When was the last time you played? Playing is physical activity without connection to the outcome. It isn't about winning or losing or how fast or slow you are. Go on a run to nowhere. Jump on a trampoline. Try to catch fireflies. Skip rope. Hit a ball against a wall with a tennis racquet. Move your body for the sake of movement. Enjoy what your body can do and tell your inner perfectionist to go fly a kite (literally!).

Now that you've silenced your inner perfectionist, you can move on to the next step of becoming fascinated with things and that's to have a novel experience.

This exercise is simple and will be unique to you. The only two requisites are:

(1) Do something you've never done before.

(2) Silence your inner perfectionist before you do it so you can enter a state of fascination.

Don't know where to begin? Here's a list of potential activities to try:

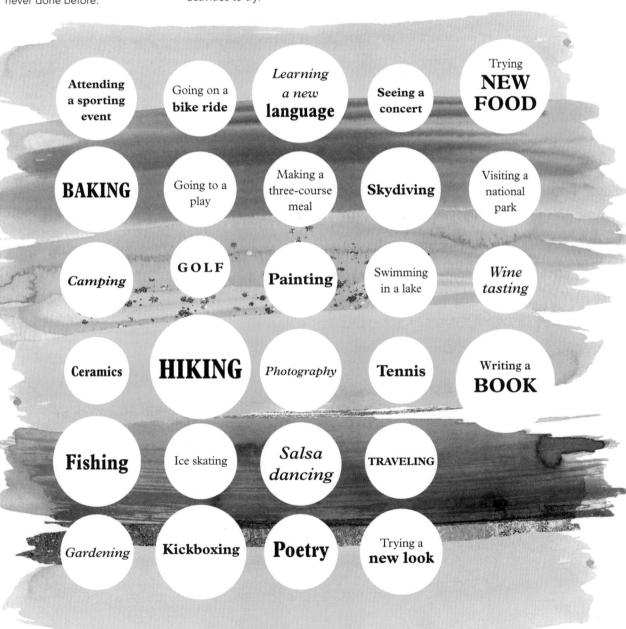

Attending a sporting event

Going on a bike ride

Learning a new language

Seeing a concert

Trying NEW FOOD

BAKING

Going to a play

Making a three-course meal

Skydiving

Visiting a national park

Camping

GOLF

Painting

Swimming in a lake

Wine tasting

Ceramics

HIKING

Photography

Tennis

Writing a BOOK

Fishing

Ice skating

Salsa dancing

TRAVELING

Gardening

Kickboxing

Poetry

Trying a new look

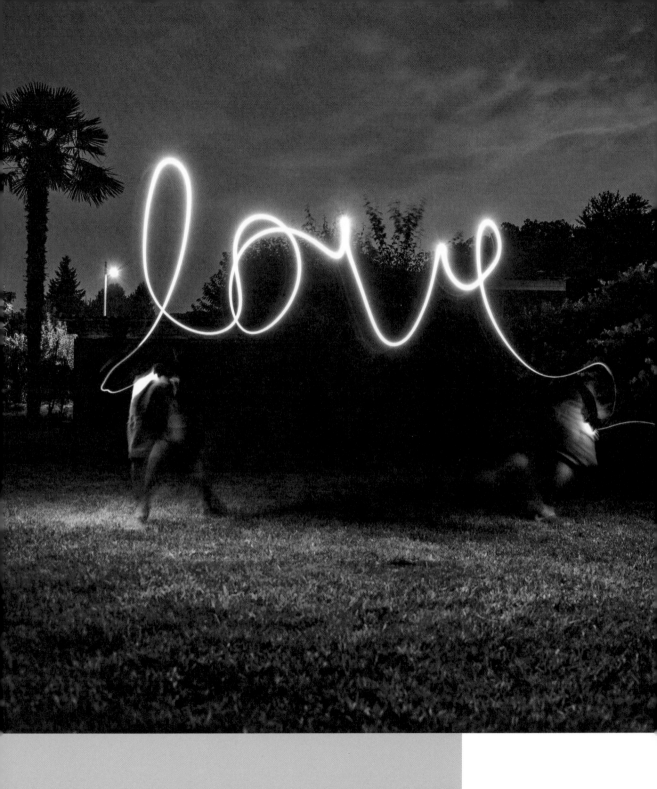

EXERCISES IN CONNECTION

The following two things can help connect you with the world: staying present and practicing active acknowledgement and gratitude.

You can truly connect with your surroundings by tapping into your senses. Refer back to the "Five Senses Exercise" (page 37). It works beautifully to bring you back to the present moment.

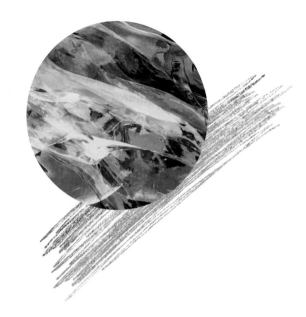

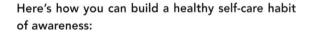

Much like a child will wave at and greet inanimate objects ("Hi, moon!" "Hi there, tree!"), you can do the same. It may seem silly at first, but you must acknowledge something before you can be grateful for it. This exercise helps you appreciate the energy in everything around you. It lets you stay connected to the space in which you exist and heightens your awareness.

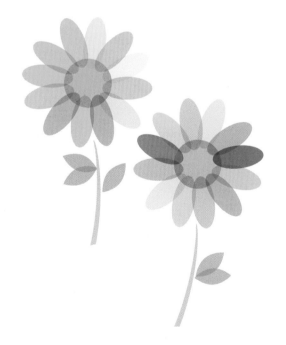

Here's how you can build a healthy self-care habit of awareness:

(1) **Mentally greet the area around you.** You can acknowledge the inanimate objects in your surroundings with the same enthusiasm you'd show when greeting a friend. Make the greeting (whether to yourself or out loud) match the way you would normally greet a person. For example, you can say:

> "Hi, garden of flowers. Great to see you!"
>
> "Hello, sun in the sky. How have you been?"

(2) **Personalize each item around you.** This helps deepen your awareness, perception, and connection to your physical environment, which in turn enhances your emotional state and sense of stability.

Efficiency

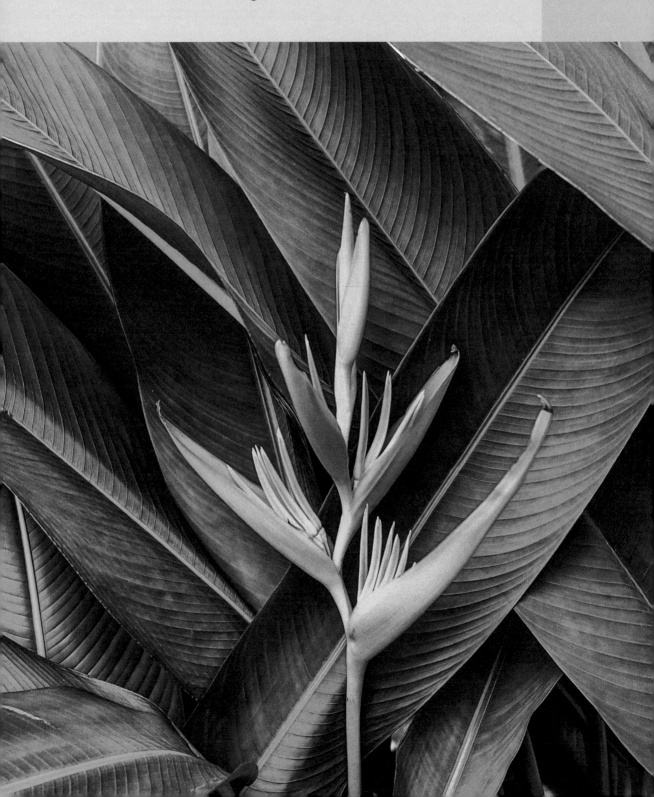

Do you wish you had more hours in the day or feel like you have way too much on your plate? Or maybe you wish life could slow down—but you know that's not always possible. These feelings can lead to general overwhelm. Luckily, you can harness a skill that will help you free up time in your day.

Time Management

It's called *efficiency*. Learning how to work with your natural rhythms can get you in sync with the flow of your day, speed up tasks, maximize productivity and, in turn, save time in your day to do the things that make you happy.

———

The key to becoming more efficient is understanding how the human brain works, identifying your flow, and blocking out your time.

THE MYTH OF MULTITASKING

Some people may brag about being master multitaskers—perhaps you've even claimed to be one. But in reality, multitasking is impossible because the human brain can only focus on one thing at time. What you're experiencing when you claim to be multitasking is actually your brain rapidly switching from one area of focus to another. This wastes valuable brain power and proves to be an inefficient way to function.[27]

In fact, multitasking trains your brain to behave poorly. Each task, regardless of how small, that you "complete" (like responding to a text message) releases dopamine, the reward hormone, in your brain. This surge of "happiness" trains your brain to jump from small task to small task just to receive more dopamine. You should fight this tendency and instead focus efficiently on a single task for the even greater reward of freeing up the time that you would have otherwise wasted while multitasking.

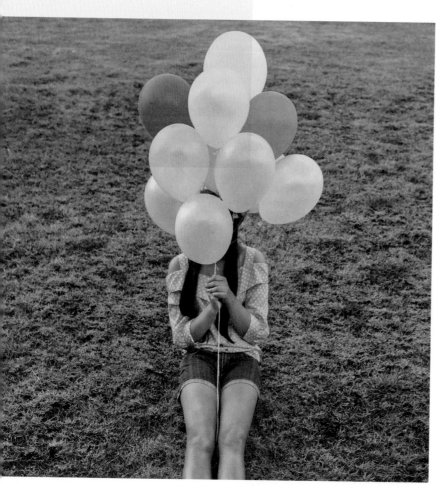

What you consider to be multitasking is harming you in the following ways:[28]

- Creates mental exhaustion so you lose valuable energy that could be used on the things you enjoy.

- Lowers the quality of your work and makes you more inefficient.

- Increases stress levels by boosting production of the stress hormone cortisol.

- Reduces productivity by 40 percent.

You can protect yourself from multitasking by:

- Only doing one task at a time.

- Silencing your phone and email inbox and only checking them at pre-determined times.

It's natural to have an energy cycle that ebbs and flows throughout the day. To figure out your general flow, you must be in sync with your unique rhythms. This simple, week-long exercise will tell you a lot about yourself and how to schedule your day.

You'll need:

Spiral-bound notebook

Pen

Watch

Directions:

(1) Each day, rate your energy levels on a scale of one to five each hour of the day (begin upon waking). A rating of one is very low energy (feeling sluggish and like you want to take a nap), and a five is very high energy (focused and productive). Keep track of this in your notebook. At the end of a day, the page in your notebook might look like this →

(2) Repeat this on a separate page in your notebook for each day of the week.

Monday

6:00 a.m. – 3

7:00 a.m. – 5

8:00 a.m. – 5

9:00 a.m. – 5

10:00 a.m. – 4

11:00 a.m. – 4

12:00 p.m. – 3

1:00 p.m. – 2

2:00 p.m. – 1

3:00 p.m. – 2

4:00 p.m. – 3

5:00 p.m. – 4

6:00 p.m. – 5

7:00 p.m. – 4

8:00 p.m. – 3

9:00 p.m. – 2

10:00 p.m. – 1

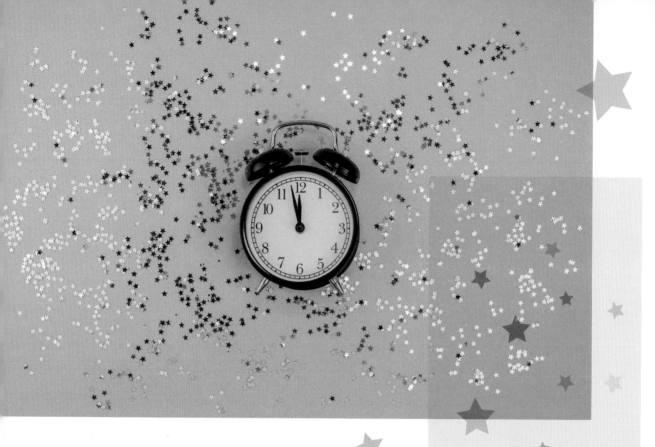

③ At the end of the week, look for general patterns in your behavior. Maybe your energy is at its peak from 7:00 a.m. to 11:00 a.m. and then again between 5 p.m. and 7 p.m. Maybe you learn that you have a ton of energy during the first half of the day and run out of steam for the remainder of the day. You might find that you're a night owl and have a surge of energy in the evenings. There's no right and wrong time to feel a burst of energy—it's just important to note your high-energy and low-energy zones.

④ Write your highest and lowest energy times down in your journal.

⑤ Create efficient time blocks of your day by scheduling important tasks that require you to focus during your high-energy periods and less urgent matters or relaxation time during your low-energy zones.

Time Blocking: Maximize Your Day to Clear Time for You

Now that you've identified your general flow, you can schedule your day by placing tasks in their appropriate time slot: do high-priority and engaging tasks during your periods of high energy and complete low-priority or low-level tasks during your periods of low energy. By doing this, you've created a time management system that works with your natural energy cycle called "time blocking."

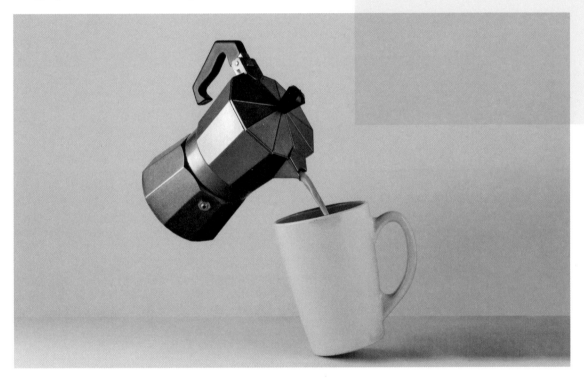

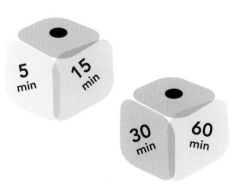

To effectively time block, you need to employ time integrity. Set aside an amount of time for a task and stick to it—giving *all of your focus* to *only* that task during a specified period of time. You can use your phone or a time cube to keep track of time. A time cube is a tabletop timer broken down into time increments of five, fifteen, thirty, and sixty minutes. This helps you mentally turn a task into a kind of beat-the-clock game.

How to Block Out Time

You'll need:

A planner (or the calendar on your phone or computer) that shows an hourly day view

A pen you love to write with (if using a planner and not a digital calendar)

A time cube (you can find one online) or the timer on your phone

(1) Make a list of things you want to complete in one given day.

(2) Now reorder that list based on order of priority (the first thing on the list should be the most important).

(3) Using the increments on a time cube (five minutes, fifteen minutes, thirty minutes, and sixty minutes) write down the amount of time needed to complete the task next to the task's name on your priority list. If a task is going to take, say, two and a half hours to complete, break it down into sections (i.e., two 60-minute sessions and one 30-minute session or six 30-minute sessions).

(4) Put the important priorities into your schedule for the first day. Plan to complete these tasks during your high-energy period. Fill in the rest of the list in the open spots in your day, making sure to match priority level with your energy level. Leave a slight buffer of time (five minutes) between tasks.

(5) Now let your day begin! When it's time to start the first task, remove all distraction. Silence your phone and turn off email notifications. Set the time cube (or the timer on your phone) for the projected time it will take to complete this task or a specific portion of it.

(6) Work on your task until the time cube alerts you that time is up.

(7) Turn the time cube (or set the timer on your phone) to five minutes. Take a break from whatever it is you're doing.

Listen to a song and dance. Drink some water or have a quick snack. All of these activities gets you out of what you're doing and gets your body moving. Adding a change to the monotony raises your endorphin levels, psychologically enforces the importance of celebration, and encourages your brain so it can remain efficient.

(8) Repeat the cycle for the next task.

(10) At the end of the day, notice how much you got done and your overall mood.

Today

SCHEDULE	TO DO
08.00	
09.00	
10.00	
11.00	
12.00	
13.00	
14.00	
15.00	
16.00	
17.00	
18.00	
19.00	

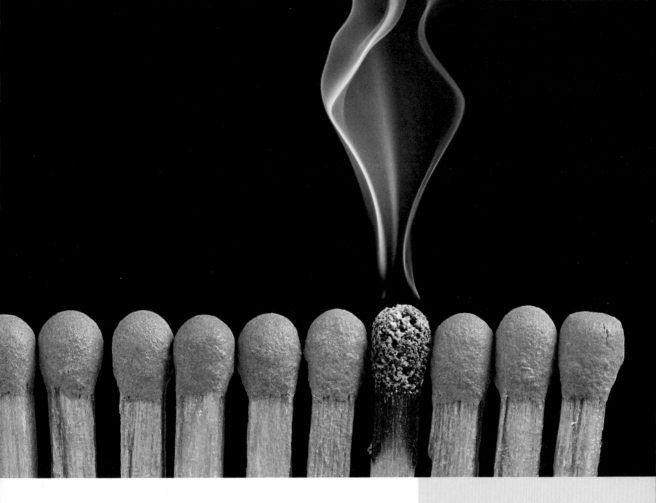

CREATING A SCHEDULE THAT PROTECTS SELF-CARE

It is important that you prioritize self-care when time blocking your day. Self-care exercises help keep you stable, happy, and balanced, which will make your day even more productive and efficient. Scheduling in breaks, allowing yourself to do "nothing" as an activity (you deserve some downtime to recharge!), and prioritizing time blocks for fun and rejuvenation will create balance and joy in your life.

Social Media

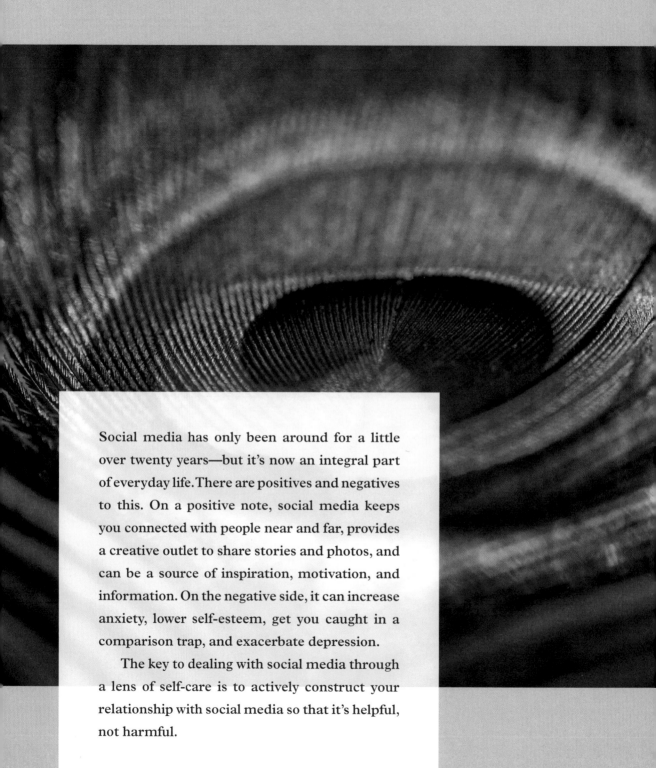

Social media has only been around for a little over twenty years—but it's now an integral part of everyday life. There are positives and negatives to this. On a positive note, social media keeps you connected with people near and far, provides a creative outlet to share stories and photos, and can be a source of inspiration, motivation, and information. On the negative side, it can increase anxiety, lower self-esteem, get you caught in a comparison trap, and exacerbate depression.

The key to dealing with social media through a lens of self-care is to actively construct your relationship with social media so that it's helpful, not harmful.

The Comparison Trap

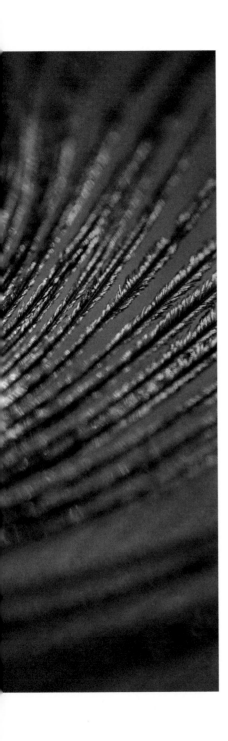

It's easy to look at someone's "life" on social media and compare your life to his or hers. You might begin to feel bad about how you look, the state of your home, your social life, your love life, or a variety of other things. If this starts to happen, remind yourself that social media is simply a highlight reel and that you're are not seeing the whole picture (or what's hiding behind those perfectly staged photos).

———

For example, the woman you think has a "flawless body" may have photoshopped her picture because in reality she doesn't love the way she looks. Or the man with the "successful career" might be suffering from anxiety, overwhelm, and exhaustion, or feel stressed that he doesn't have time for his family.

The family with the "dream kitchen" might have a pile of toys and a screaming baby in another room of their house. Perhaps they are in major debt from home renovations, or maybe they inherited the money to pay for it. You never truly know another person's story—so there's no point in comparing your reality to someone else's life.

Granted, what's happening behind the scenes isn't always negative; these people may have happy, stable, balanced lives—but they're also human (therefore not perfect). But if you can't enjoy social media for what it is—that is, a mere glimpse into someone else's life—and you're constantly comparing yourself to others to the point of feeling envious, insecure, or hopeless, it's time to take matters into your own hands.

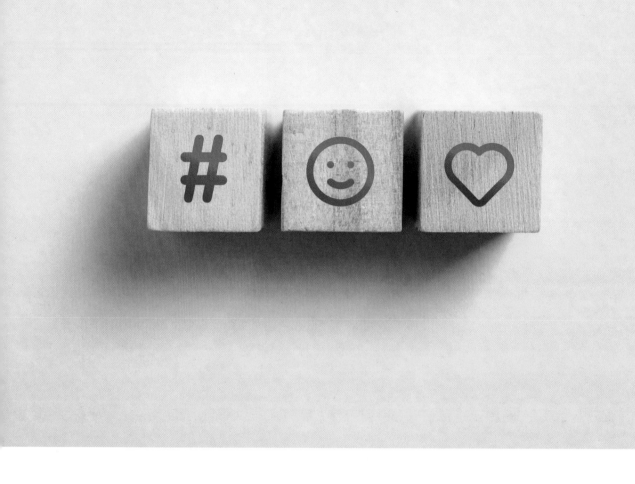

Social Media Curation

The best way to use social media is to connect with friends (old and new), inspire others and be inspired, and find beauty and motivation. Social media can boost your mood if you carefully curate your content. Think of your social media account as a museum. Anyone you follow can "post" their art to your museum walls. Is their "art," consisting of photos, opinions, videos, words, and energy, the kind you want to look at? Is it the kind of art you would allow in your "museum?"

Ask this question about each person you follow.

- **If the answer is YES:** Continue to follow and interact with this person and be grateful for the beauty and motivation that they provide.

- **If the answer is NO:** For your own mental self-care, you should unfollow, block, or censor these "artists."

Limiting Screen Time

A good way to monitor your social media consumption is by setting clearly defined screen limits for yourself each day. Once these screen limits are in place, you can schedule them into your day so that you can control your social media interactions (and not the other way around).

Think about your social media needs. For most people, twenty minutes a day is more than enough. Give yourself ten minutes in the morning and ten minutes in the evening to check social media. Set a timer for the allotted amount of time before opening social media and then close it the second the timer goes off.

Soon enough you'll have control over your relationship with social media so that it doesn't take over other areas of your life.

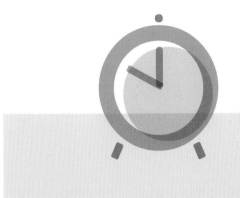

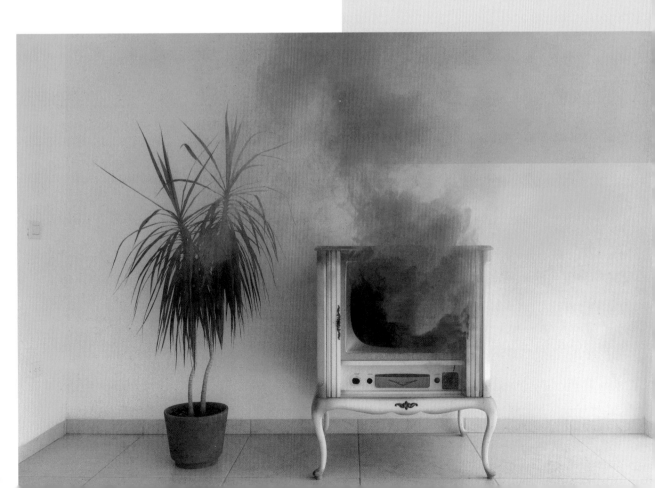

Social Media Detox

If you find that curating your social media and setting screen time limits still doesn't eradicate your feelings of envy, poor self-image, or anxiety (or if you think you have a social media addiction), it's in your best interest to commit to a social media detox. This break will help reset your mind and your perspective.

Signs that you may need a social media detox:

- You find yourself checking your phone numerous times an hour to see if there are any new posts or if you have new likes or comments.
- You feel anxious after you look at social media—and you feel anxious if you go too long without checking it.
- You feel worse about yourself after scrolling through pictures and posts on social media.
- You find yourself losing valuable time during the day because you're on social media.
- Your world view becomes more self-centered after looking through social media.
- You believe that all of the images you see on social media are reality.

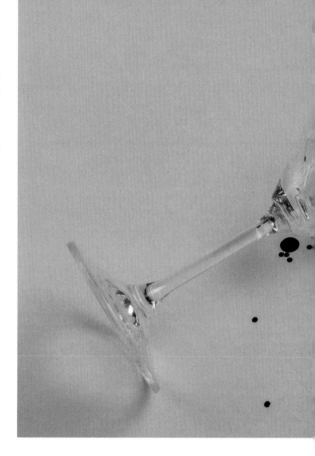

A social media detox is when you remove social media from your daily life for a set period of time. If you're truly addicted, going cold turkey may prove too difficult. In this case, you may need to start with stepping away for a few hours at a time until you can work your way up to eliminating social media for a day or more.

This addiction is caused by dopamine. This reward hormone in your brain triggers every time you get a like, message, comment, or any other type of interaction on social media. Dopamine trains your brain to become addicted to this cycle of cause (you post a picture) and effect (someone likes it). Shockingly, it takes approximately one hundred days for dopamine levels to return to normal.[29]

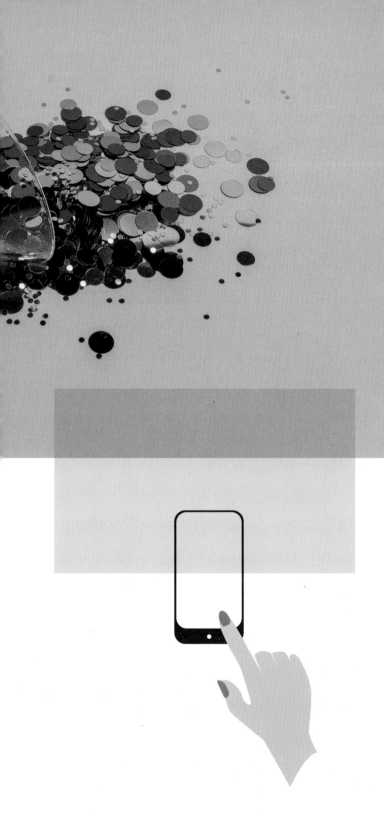

Social Media Detox Exercise

You should start with a few hours of no social media, giving yourself time to work up to a day, then a week, and eventually a month. After this detox, you may decide to forgo social media completely or you may find that after some time away, you now have a healthier grasp on it.

(1) **Commit to a set amount of time you won't look at your account.** If you're limiting this to a day or less, skip to the next step. But if you want to detox for longer than a day, deactivate (but do not erase) your accounts and remove the apps from your phone.

(2) **Every time you have the urge to look at your social media, busy yourself with another self-care exercise.** Go for a walk. Get your nails done with a friend. Take a bath. Try any of the self-care exercises in this book.

(3) **At the end of each day of the detox (it may only be one day at first), write down how you felt stepping away from social media and what you did with your free time.** This will provide your brain with positive affirmations—reaffirming the fact that it's beneficial to use social media less frequently.

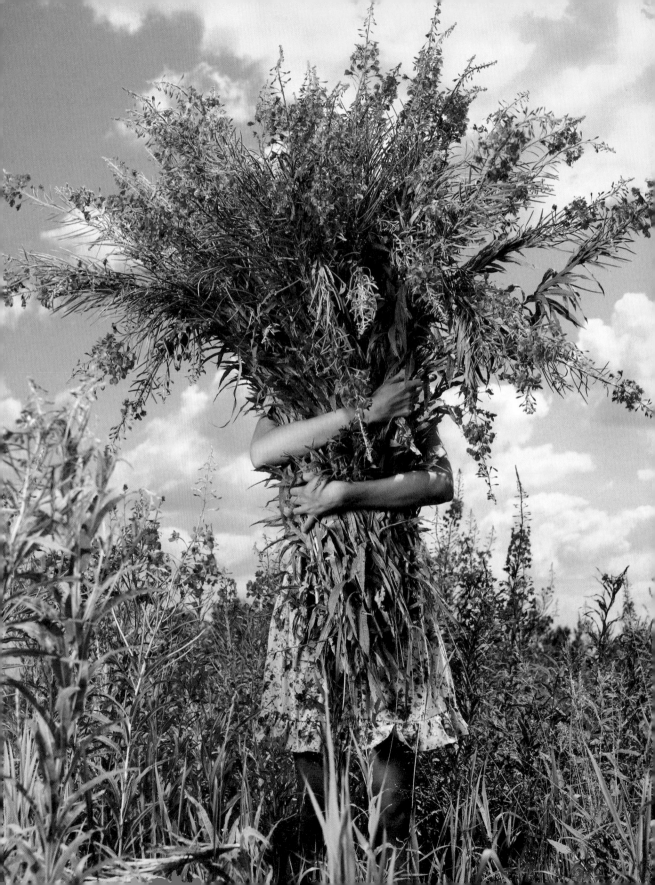

3

EMOTIONAL SELF-CARE

*"When we self-regulate well,
we are better able to control the
trajectory of our emotional lives and
resulting actions based on our values
and sense of purpose."*

—AMY LEIGH MERCREE

Self-Love

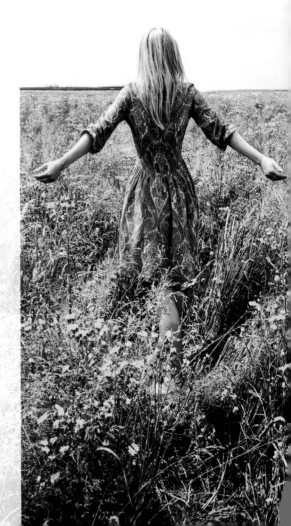

Love. It's something we all seek, and yet there's a tremendous amount of confusion surrounding the concept.

We're inundated with ideas of what love is supposed to be. Books, movies, "reality" television shows, societal pressures, the media, advertisements— the list goes on and on. We receive images of what love is supposed to look and feel like—but these are only confusing and unrealistic distractions that will keep you from finding the kind of genuine love you desire.

There's only one definition of love that truly matters: the one you define within yourself. To figure this out, you have to do the work. You have to take a deep dive into who you are and relentlessly pursue yourself with a fervent passion.

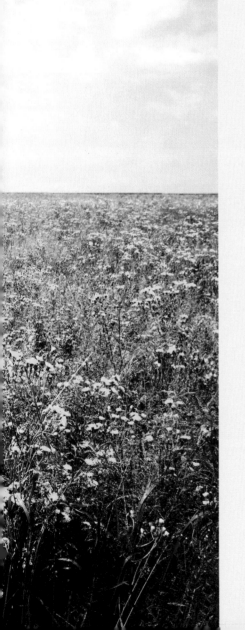

Do you love yourself? Do you show yourself care, empathy, kindness, and understanding? Do you find yourself thrilling, exciting, astonishing, and captivating? This type of self-love comes first—love yourself and the rest will follow.

———

Self-love might sound like a radical concept, but it's not. It's simply taking the love, attention, affection, forgiveness, happiness, acceptance, and joy that you give to others and turning it inward *before* giving your love away.

If you're like most people, you probably don't love yourself completely yet. But the good news is, this kind of love can be learned. Even better news: self-love is the ultimate form of self-care.

When you learn how to love yourself it becomes easier to attract the right kind of love (platonic and romantic) into your life, set clear boundaries because you know your worth, love someone else without being co-dependent, make decisions that align with who you are, and achieve internal emotional stability.

This steadfast self-love will permeate into all areas of your life. The result: a life you love as much as you love yourself.

How do you learn to love yourself? The activities in this section will help you achieve an everlasting self-love. And if the love you have for yourself should ever waver, simply repeat these exercises at any time to reignite the spark.

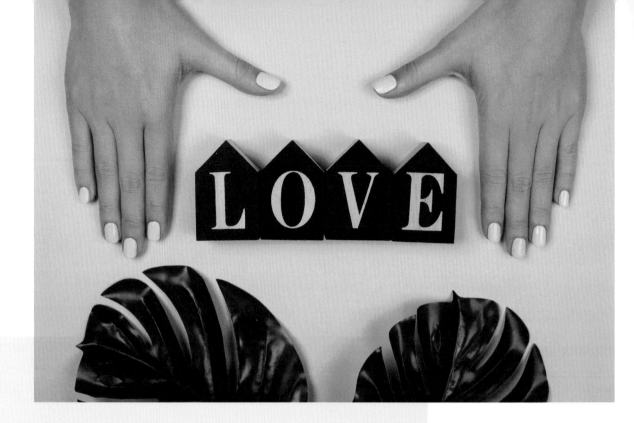

Affirmations

An affirmation is a positive thought or statement, written or spoken, that challenges self-limiting beliefs and replaces patterns of negative thinking with patterns of positive thinking. When you consistently and repetitively implement affirmations into your life, you will improve your mood, train your mind to choose positive thoughts over negative ones, boost your confidence, and elevate your outlook.

A positive view of yourself is the first step toward self-love. You receive countless messages daily—directly and subliminally—telling you that you're not good enough. You need to be perfect to be loved. True love is reserved for the lucky. These messages only serve to feed the negative voice inside of your head that says: "You're good enough. You need to be better. You need to be perfect because that's the only way you deserve love."

To demonstrate that this idea is false, think of this: Are the people in your life that you love perfect? No. They're not—and still, you love them. You love them because you recognize all of the positive things about them and tend to focus on these things in spite of their imperfections. You deserve to love yourself with the same commitment and focus on positivity—but first you must gain control over the negative voice in your head telling you that you're not worthy of love.

To silence this negative self-talk, you have to actively replace negative thoughts with positive ones. This trains your brain to choose the positive over the negative. Essentially, you must combat the negativity that you've been unknowingly absorbing throughout your life.

How do you do this? An easy way to rewire your self-talk is through positive daily affirmations.

Replacing Negative Thoughts With Positive Affirmations

(1) **Identify your predominant negative thoughts.** Take a piece of paper and draw a line down the center of the page lengthwise. In the left column, make a list of the things you either don't like about yourself or think you need to change about yourself. This part of the exercise may be a bit painful, but it's necessary to identify your pain points so you can eliminate them.

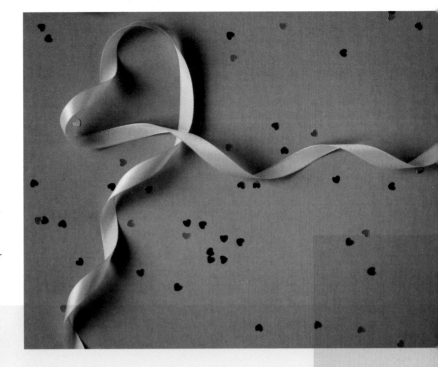

(2) **Replace your negative self-talk with positive affirmations.** Now you can begin to rewire your thinking. In the right column, write a positive thought that counters the negative one. Think of it like an argument: your brain is telling you one thing, and now you're going to tell your brain that it's wrong. Perhaps your negative self-talk consists of a nasty voice in your head saying, "You're too stupid to be taken seriously." Write that statement in the left column. Then in the right column, fight back against the phrase in the left column in your own powerful voice. You can write something like, "I am smart and capable, and my opinion is important." Or you can write, "My mind is unique, and I see the world in a remarkable way. I am intelligent and valuable." Write anything that feels like something you would want someone else to say to you to make you feel loved.

(3) **Cut the paper in half lengthwise and get rid of the left-hand column.** It's time to symbolically say good riddance to all of the negativity that's been clouding your thinking. You may choose to throw this half away, tear it into little pieces, burn it, toss it in the ocean— you get the idea. Get rid of it in a way that tells your brain that negative thinking will no longer be tolerated.

(4) **Use the remaining statements as affirmations.** This is explained in detail in the following section on how to use affirmations.

If the previous exercise seems too daunting, you can try the following positive affirmations:

My **HEART** is full of love and goodness.

I trust myself to make great **decisions.**

I am strong and capable.

I am beautiful, radiant, and **bright.**

My mind is **LIMITLESS.**

I am **worthy** of love, capable of receiving love, and give love freely.

I have endless **energy** and use it effectively.

I am healthy, able, and live a **life** of abundance.

My **CREATIVITY** is boundless, and I have endless ideas.

I love every inch of my **BODY** and am grateful for its abilities.

LOVE flows to me and through me with ease.

I am **brave,** and I choose to be the architect of my life.

I am unique, **special,** and remarkable.

I am so **GRATEFUL** that I am me.

I love myself **DEEPLY,** unconditionally, completely, and fully.

I trust that the **FUTURE** is full of exciting opportunities and adventures.

HOW TO USE AFFIRMATIONS

These exercises can be done using numerous affirmations, or you can choose one to focus on if you want. Your affirmations can be from your own list, the sample options, or any affirmation that resonates with you.

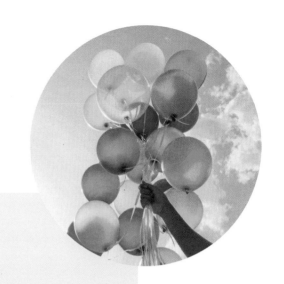

Speak it. Say the affirmation out loud confidently and with conviction. Do this five times each morning and evening.

Write it. Get a spiral notebook with lined paper. Write your affirmation over and over again on each line. Continue writing the affirmation until the page is full.

Post it. Write your affirmation on sticky notes and put them places where you're sure to see them. Good spots include: the bathroom mirror, your car dashboard, the refrigerator, your morning coffee mug (bonus points for getting your affirmation printed on a mug), your underwear drawer, your toothbrush holder.

Hear it. Record yourself saying the affirmation over and over again in a strong and clear voice. Play the recording back when you're sitting in silence or driving in your car.

See it. This is just like "speak it," but you also look yourself in the eye confidently and lovingly in the mirror as you say the affirmation.

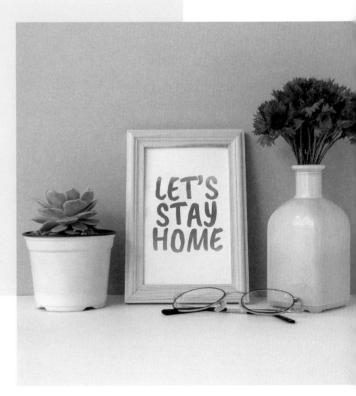

If you do these exercises every day, your positive affirmation will effectively replace negative self-talk, boost your mood, increase self-esteem, make you more self-aware, and empower you to see that you have considerable control over your thoughts.

Ritual

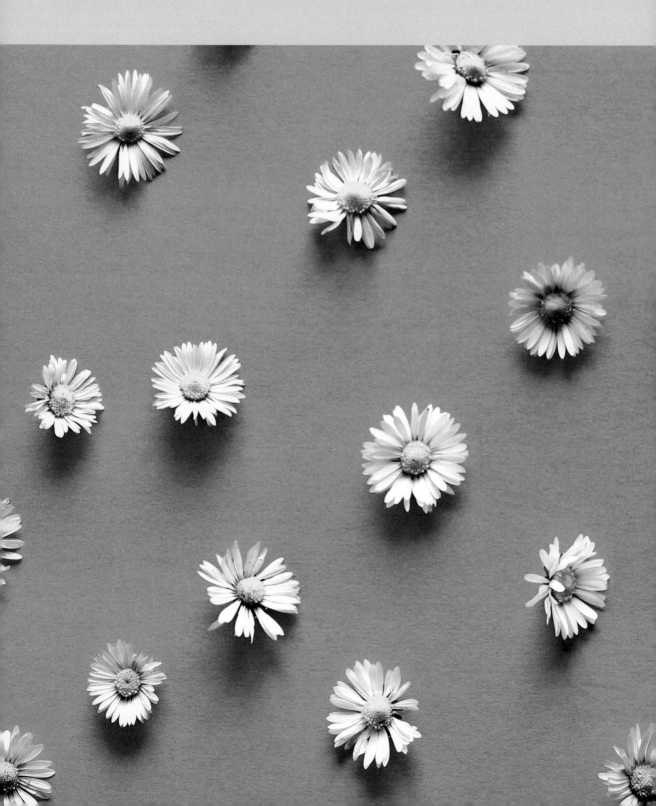

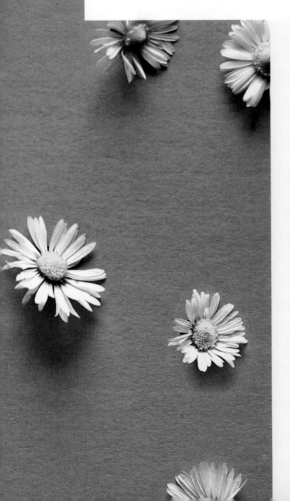

When you introduce the concept of a morning and evening ritual into your daily life, you give yourself a healthy routine that frames your day. Repetition is the key to shifting your emotional state to one of stability, clarity, calm, and satisfaction.

Morning Ritual

If you can carve out thirty minutes for yourself in the morning (even twenty will do!), you can implement a mood-boosting, focus-shifting, energy-boosting ritual at the very start of your day. You'll find that having a morning ritual sets the tone for the rest of the day. It will also help you feel happier, calm, more productive—an all-around better version of wonderful you.

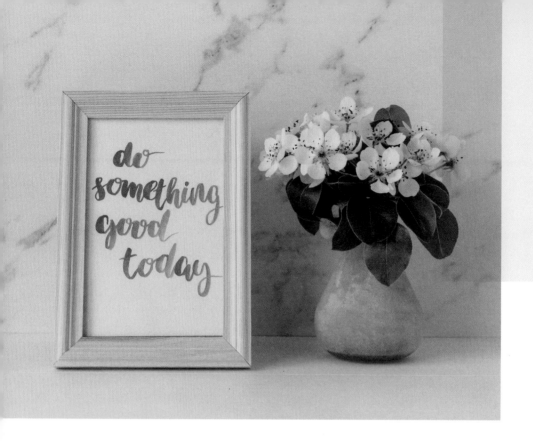

THE FIVE SIMPLE STEPS OF A MORNING RITUAL

(1) **Stretch first thing in the morning.** While you sleep, you can twist and turn in ways that can make your body feel stiff throughout the day. Stretching when you wake up puts your body back into alignment. For a series of stretches, refer to page 23.

(2) **Mediate.** Reaching a place of calm and centered clarity first thing in the morning is a beautiful way to get ahead of anything the day may throw your way. For a guide to meditation, refer to page 142.

(3) **Have a morning beverage.** Since you become dehydrated while you sleep, your body, organs, and mind need hydration to function at their highest level. For delicious and effective morning beverages, refer to page 41.

(4) **Read your morning pages.** Looking over your objectives for the day helps shift your mindset to one of gratitude and clarity. A positive outlook will make your day exponentially better. For a morning pages exercise, refer to page 78.

(5) **Do your morning skincare routine.** Taking time to care for your skin is good for your overall health and appearance. For a step-by-step skincare routine, refer to page 52.

Evening Ritual

Giving yourself another twenty to thirty minutes in the evening is the right amount of time to slow down, soothe yourself, and feel grateful. An evening routine gives you time to process the events of your day and express gratitude, which as we know helps reduce depression and prepares you for a more restful night of sleep.

THE FIVE SOOTHING STEPS OF AN EVENING RITUAL

1. **Stretch before bed.** Engaging in slow stretches sends a signal to your body that it is time to prepare for rest. For a series of stretches, refer to page 22.

2. **Have a soothing beverage.** A warm, nourishing beverage prepares your digestive system and body for rest. For a soothing evening drink, refer to Golden Milk beverage on page 41.

3. **Do your evening skincare routine.** It's important to fall asleep with a clean face and nourished skin to help fight breakouts and signs of aging. For a simple skincare routine, refer to page 52.

4. **Write in your gratitude journal.** Reminding yourself of the good things in your life leads to a more peaceful, deeper sleep. For gratitude journal basics, refer to page 81.

5. **Meditate.** A meditation practice before bed sends a signal to your brain to relax, prepare for rest, and release any emotional pain or anxiety from the day. For a guide to meditation, refer to page 142.

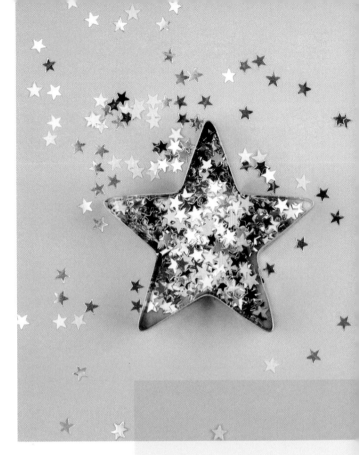

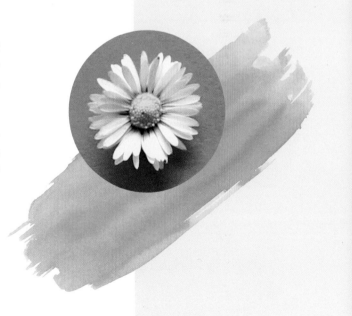

Boundaries

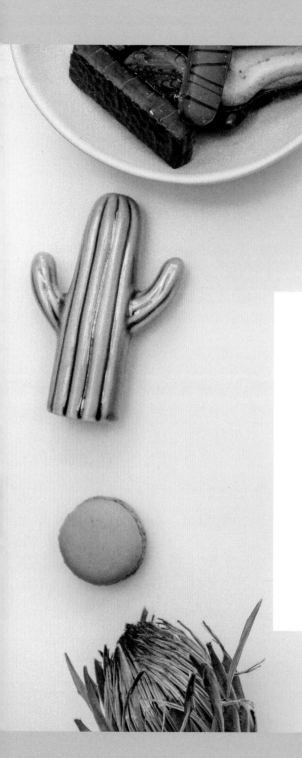

A boundary is the line you draw for yourself as to what you will and will not accept in your life. A boundary can be physical, mental, emotional, or spiritual.

Setting healthy boundaries is imperative to having control and ownership over your life and your happiness. When you begin to allow other people to infringe upon your value system, you may feel depressed, anxious, or spread too thin.

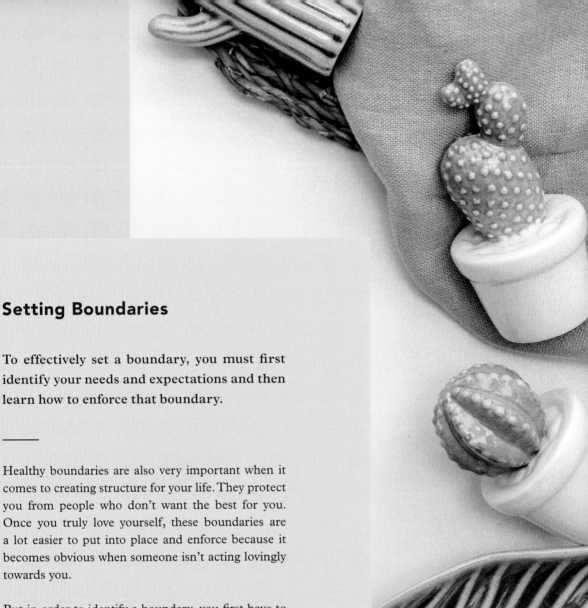

Setting Boundaries

To effectively set a boundary, you must first identify your needs and expectations and then learn how to enforce that boundary.

———

Healthy boundaries are also very important when it comes to creating structure for your life. They protect you from people who don't want the best for you. Once you truly love yourself, these boundaries are a lot easier to put into place and enforce because it becomes obvious when someone isn't acting lovingly towards you.

But in order to identify a boundary, you first have to believe the following statement: "I deserve respect." Once you accept that you deserve respect, your boundaries will be clear. The following exercise can help solidify them for you.

Identifying Your Boundries

You'll need:

Two blank sheets of paper

A pen you love to write with

① Take out a piece of paper and fold it in half lengthwise. Unfold the paper.

② Title the top of the left-hand column SAFE.

③ Title the top of the right-hand column UNSAFE.

④ On the left-hand side, make a list of all of the things in your life that *make you feel safe.* Examples include:

- Your favorite people who make you feel emotionally safe.

- A movie that gets you to your "good place."

- A song or genre that resonates with you.

- Types of clothing that you like to wear.

- An amount of money that makes you feel financially secure.

- The kind of home/shelter that makes you feel safe.

- Free time that lets you be yourself.

You can add to this list. There's no right or wrong thing seeing as this list is unique to you.

⑤ On the right-hand side, make a list of all of the things in your life that *make you feel unsafe.* This side may be emotionally difficult to write. You can include:

- Traumas

- Things that make you feel disrespected

- Things you don't like

- Values that go against your own

Include anything that threatens your sense of self on this list.

⑥ When you assess these lists side-by-side, the boundaries that suit your life should become clear.

For example:

You wrote that your home makes you feel secure on the SAFE side. On the UNSAFE side, you wrote that you don't feel safe when someone drops by your home announced. One of your boundaries would be: "I need people to give me advance notice (define the amount of notice you need specifically) before visiting the space I feel is my sanctuary."

Here's another example:

You wrote that being surrounded by friends that you know love you makes you feel safe on the SAFE side. On the UNSAFE side, you wrote that you don't feel safe when you don't know how someone feels about you. One of your boundaries would be: "I only spend time with the people who express their intentions and feelings about me, making me feel confident and safe in their love for me."

⑦ Now pull out the second sheet of paper and title it, MY BOUNDARIES. Write all identified boundaries on this paper.

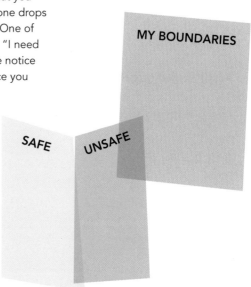

Saying "No"

Now that you've identified your boundaries, it's up to you to make sure that they're not violated. But if a boundary is violated after you've clearly expressed it to someone, you must protect yourself by enforcing your own boundary. To enforce a boundary, you must believe the following words:

"I demand respect."

This can be difficult because many people are programmed by society to be "people pleasers." If you love and respect yourself, the first person you should be pleasing—above all others—is you. If you are the person who's not happy with a situation, it's likely that one of your boundaries is being violated. There's also a chance that feeling violated or disrespected could alert you to a boundary you didn't know you needed or trigger an awareness that one of your pre-identified boundaries is being crossed. Remember, when you feel threatened, one of your boundaries is being tested.

Once you realize that your boundary is being pushed, here are steps to reinforce it:

① Learn how to say "no." There is a lot of power in this word—perhaps it's this power that makes many people afraid to use it because they're worried about how other people will view them. People who truly respect you will understand that when you politely say "no" to something in order to enforce one of your boundaries that you are coming from a place of self-love and self-respect. If they can't see it this way, it means one of two things:

- They haven't done their own personal development work to foster self-love and self-respect, which essentially makes them incapable of recognizing and respecting others' boundaries.

- They don't respect you, your boundaries, your time, or your value system.

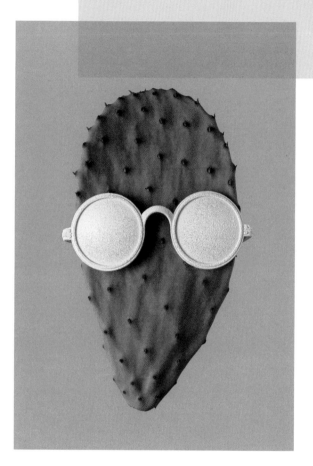

② You must enforce your "no." If someone doesn't honor or respect you after you've clearly communicated your boundaries, you must remove yourself from the toxic situation. You can do this by physically leaving, verbally asserting that you won't accept this behavior and will leave if it doesn't change, or end the relationship. All of those solutions may be difficult in the moment, but they'll serve you in the long run and help your life continue on the trajectory you desire and deserve.

Mindset

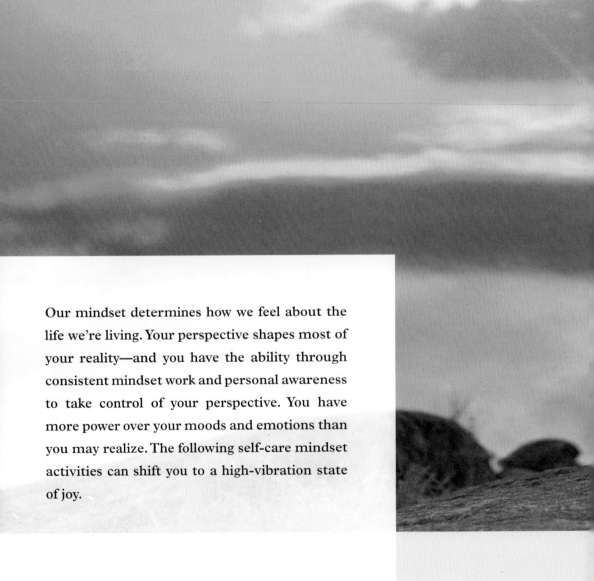

Our mindset determines how we feel about the life we're living. Your perspective shapes most of your reality—and you have the ability through consistent mindset work and personal awareness to take control of your perspective. You have more power over your moods and emotions than you may realize. The following self-care mindset activities can shift you to a high-vibration state of joy.

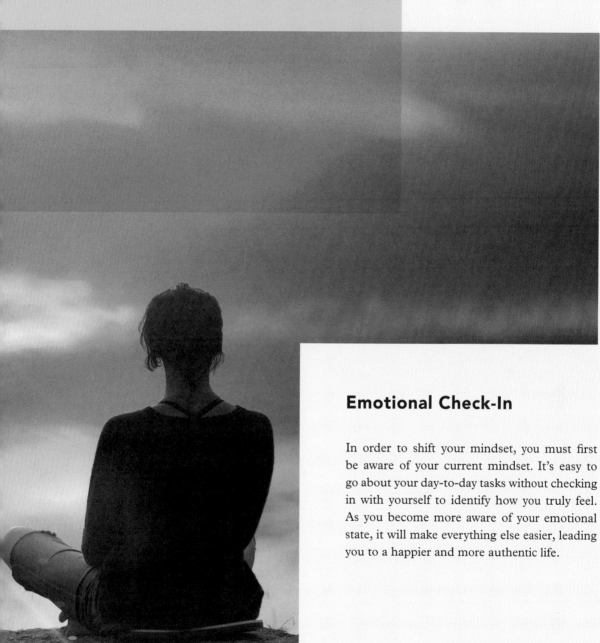

Emotional Check-In

In order to shift your mindset, you must first be aware of your current mindset. It's easy to go about your day-to-day tasks without checking in with yourself to identify how you truly feel. As you become more aware of your emotional state, it will make everything else easier, leading you to a happier and more authentic life.

How to Check in With Your Emotions

You'll need:

Phone with a timer or alarm

Notebook

A pen you love to write with

(1) Every day for a week, set an alert on your phone to go off every two hours from the time you wake up to the time you go to sleep.

(2) Each time the alarm goes off, pause and reflect. How do you feel in this moment? What emotions are you experiencing? Are you feeling:

- Grumpy?
- Anxious?
- Happy?
- Excited?
- Sad?
- Joyful?

You can list more than one emotion because it's human nature to experience a variety of feelings simultaneously.

(3) After you check in with yourself, write down the time and what you were feeling in your notebook.

(4) Each day, use a fresh sheet in your notebook to capture your feelings.

(5) At the end of the week, look at your moods. You may notice a pattern; perhaps your mood shifts during a certain time of the day. Or maybe your moods are all over the place and a bit unpredictable. This will help you better understand your mood shifts and swings, giving you an emotional baseline from which to base a range of emotions.

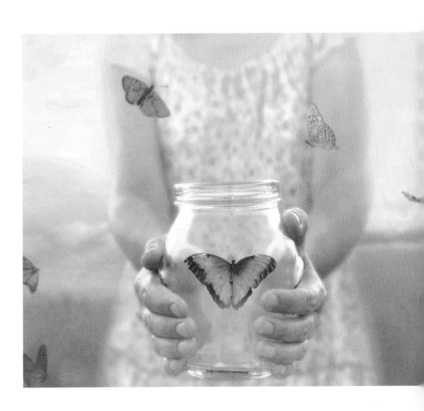

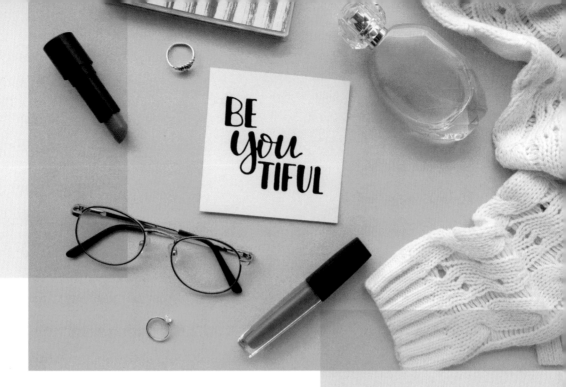

Shift to Happy: Mirror Exercise

If you commit to this two-minute exercise every day for a month, you'll notice an increase in your happiness. Two minutes a day for only thirty days is equivalent to one hour a month, yet it can make a massive difference in your overall joy.

Based on science, the simple exercise below psychologically tricks your brain into releasing endorphins so you'll be noticeably happier than you were only two minutes earlier due to a flood of endorphins that produce a happy state. At the end of the month, you will have effectively made your happiness a habit because it only takes twenty-eight days to make something habitual.

You'll need:

A mirror

1. After you wake up, head straight to a mirror and set a two-minute timer.

2. Make eye contact with yourself in the mirror. Smile broadly at yourself—not a small smile but a huge grin. Now hold that grin for two minutes. Don't worry, it's normal to feel ridiculous at first.

3. As the minutes tick on, you'll feel less ridiculous and notice yourself getting happier.

4. After two minutes, take note of the general uptick in your happiness.

TIP!

This exercise can be repeated throughout the day whenever you need a happiness boost.

"You" Time

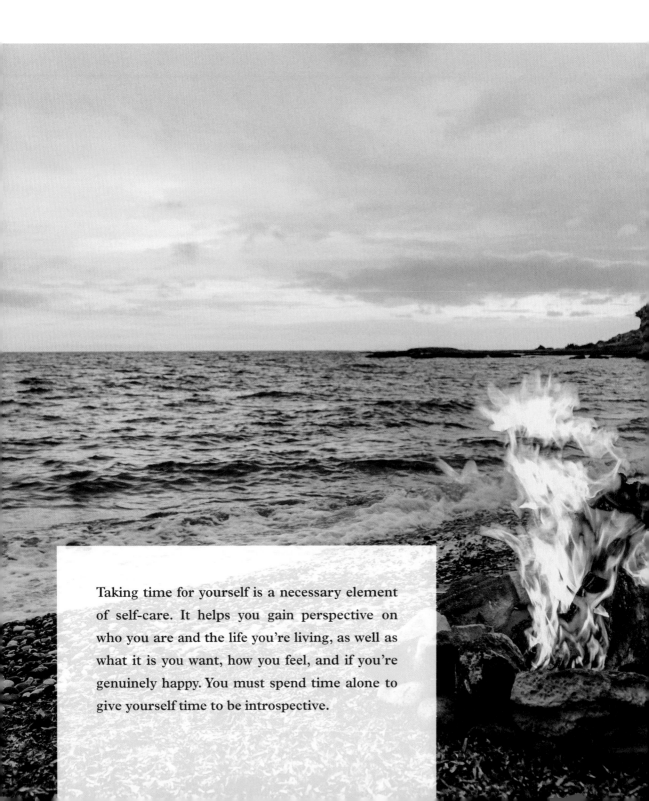

Taking time for yourself is a necessary element of self-care. It helps you gain perspective on who you are and the life you're living, as well as what it is you want, how you feel, and if you're genuinely happy. You must spend time alone to give yourself time to be introspective.

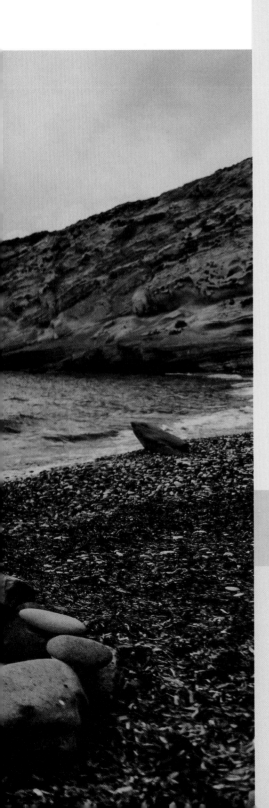

Staycation

It's human nature to take things for granted, but to stay in your happy zone, you need to remain aware and grateful for your surroundings.

———

The easiest thing to take for granted—because it can become a backdrop for your routine—is your home. Everything you see every day can go from beautiful to commonplace quickly.

To reset your mindset, take a staycation. A staycation is essentially a vacation where you stay in your own town. Seeing where you live through the eyes of a tourist or a visitor will help re-awaken your appreciation for all of the magic that is right in your backyard.

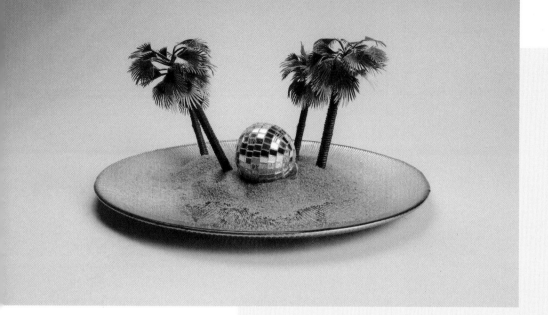

Recipe for a Mental Getaway

STEP ONE: Pick a hotel, motel, or place to stay in your town. If your town isn't tourist-friendly, choose a neighboring city or town within a thirty-minute drive. Book yourself an overnight stay.

STEP TWO: Pack an overnight bag with the following items: outfits, pajamas, and loungewear—anything that makes you feel beautiful. Put in the effort to dress the part on your staycation.

STEP THREE: When you arrive, pretend you know nothing about the town. Ask the staff at the hotel for recommendations of where to go and what to do and take their suggestions like a tourist would. Go sightseeing. Go out to dinner. Go for a walk on a beach.

Visit an art gallery or museum. Get a morning coffee at a cute café or order breakfast in bed. Most importantly, take pictures of everything!

STEP FOUR: Notice how you perceive your surroundings with fresh eyes. Are there things you've never noticed before? Anything you want to tell friends about? Did you learn anything new about yourself? Plan to take another staycation whenever you need to reset your body and mind.

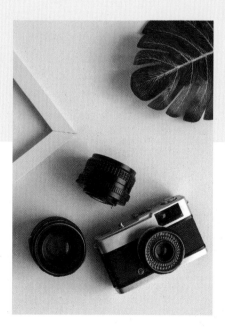

The Cycle of Introspection and Connection

Balance can be a difficult thing to identify when it comes to how you spend your time, but the concepts of *introspection* and *connection* can help keep you balanced.

Plato said, "The unexamined life is not worth living." His statement reveals the importance of introspection: if you don't examine your life, your motivations, purpose, drives, and passions, then are you truly living your life? And are you doing something worthwhile?

Introspection means taking time to check in with yourself. We live in a fast-paced society, and if you don't take time to slow down and be alone, then you won't be cognizant of the life you're living. Through self-reflection, you stop life from happening *to* you and become a more engaged participant in the game of life.

You should talk to yourself every day, multiple times a day. After you check in with yourself, write down some of your thoughts so that the conversation you had with yourself becomes tangible.

After being introspective, you have to balance this alone time with connection. This is all about reaching outside of yourself to connect with others and be in tune with what's going on around you.

If you don't balance introspection and connection, you'll feel it. For example, if you're too introspective and don't connect with people enough, you'll feel something akin to depression. And if you have too much connection without introspection, you'll experience feelings of anxiety or like you're living an inauthentic or purposeless life. When the two are in balance, you'll feel like you're living a happy and authentic life—in essence, a life with meaning.

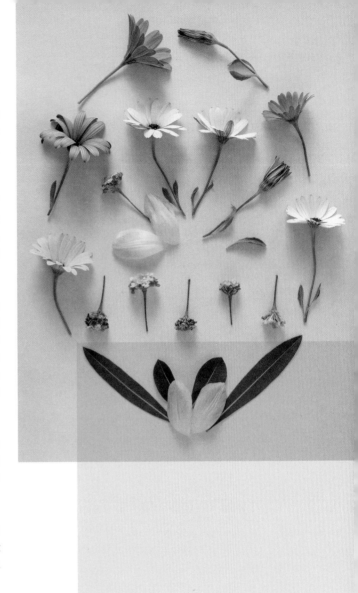

You can begin to implement this by practicing your morning routine, which involves introspection and scheduling in something social for later in the day. Bonus points if your social connection involves doing something kind for someone else.

The Cycle of Celebration

In our fast-paced, achievement-based society, it's easy to get caught in a cycle: set a goal, achieve the goal, and then immediately set another goal. Being motivated is wonderful, but if you don't acknowledge and celebrate your achievements, you could be heading for burnout or overwhelm, or perhaps you already feel this way.

The goal-achievement-goal cycle above is missing the step of celebration. Here's what your new cycle—with self-care in mind—should look like:

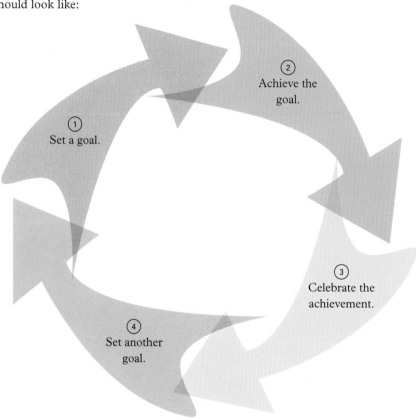

1. Set a goal.
2. Achieve the goal.
3. Celebrate the achievement.
4. Set another goal.

This cycle allows you to keep moving forward in life, growing, and progressing. But it also allows you to enjoy the fruits of your labor, stay present, feel a sense of pride in your achievements (you deserve to feel good about the things you accomplish!), and recharge before tackling the next goal.

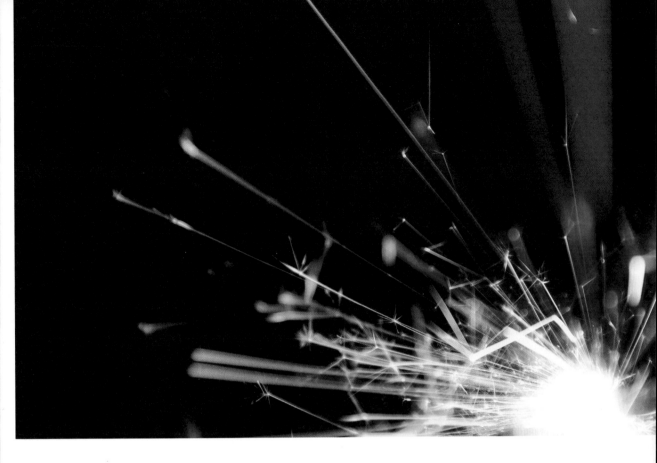

The way you celebrate is entirely up to you because different things feel good for different people. Here's a list of celebratory suggestions to help get you started:

Do anything your heart desires. The important thing is that you recognize you're celebrating something that you deserve. Now you can move on to the next goal!

- Go out to a nice dinner.
- Pour yourself a glass of champagne.
- Clap, cheer, and dance.
- Get your nails done.
- Take a trip.
- Meet friends out for happy hour.
- Go camping.
- Take a day off to relax.
- Grab coffee with your family.

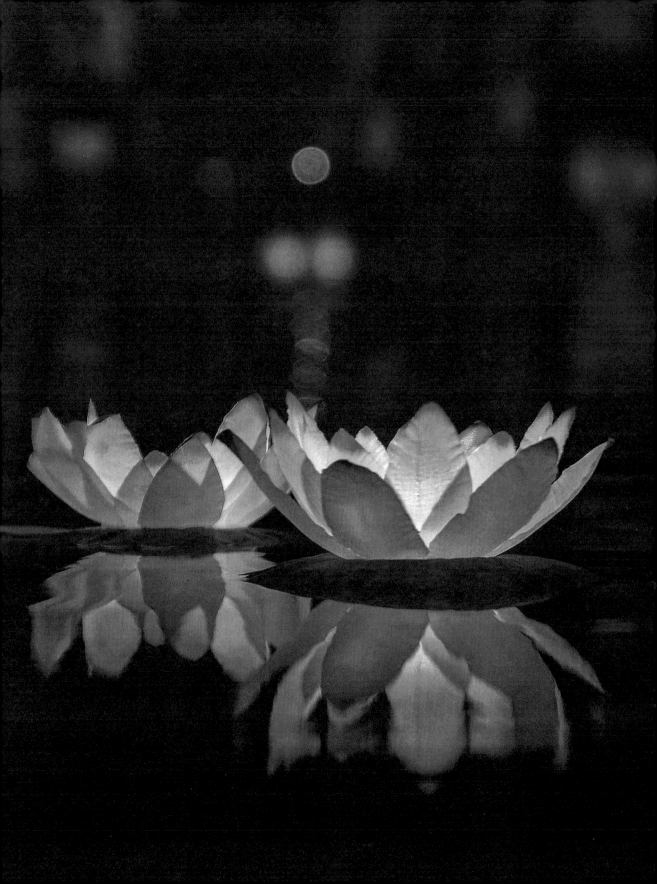

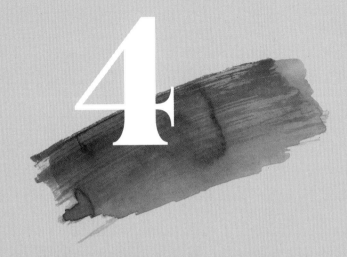

4

SPIRITUAL SELF-CARE

*"At the center of your being,
you have the answer; you know
who you are and you know
what you want."*

—LAO TZU

Meditation

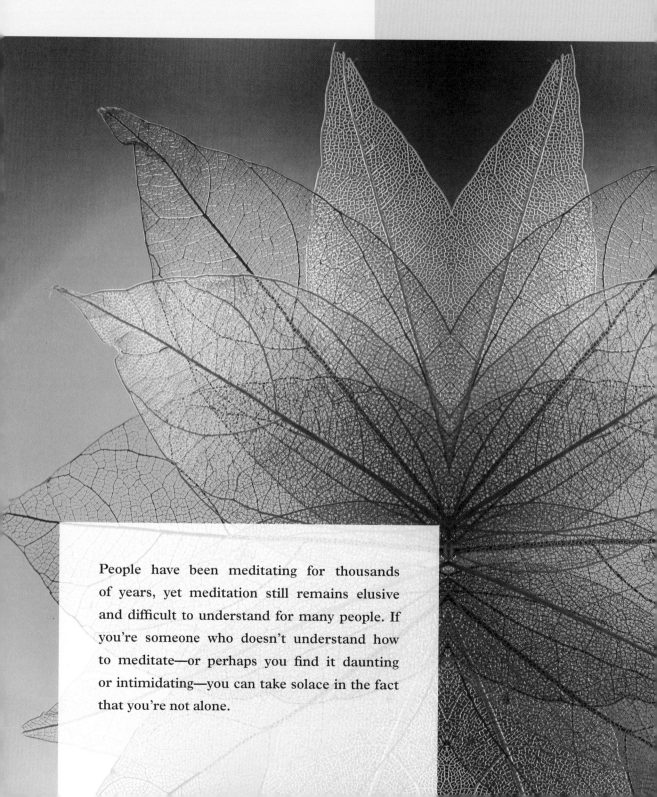

People have been meditating for thousands of years, yet meditation still remains elusive and difficult to understand for many people. If you're someone who doesn't understand how to meditate—or perhaps you find it daunting or intimidating—you can take solace in the fact that you're not alone.

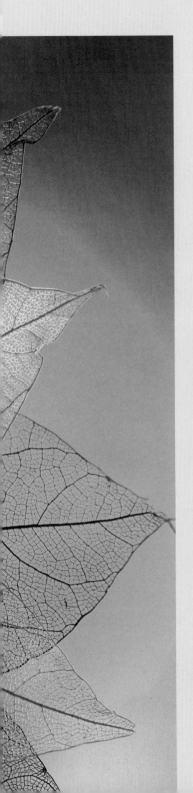

Many people give up on meditation, or refuse to begin in the first place, because they assume that the point of meditation is an "absence of thought." But that's an incorrect assumption—and it's virtually impossible.

———

Meditation is not about having a completely clear or empty mind. At its essence, meditation is an acknowledgement of the thoughts that arise while you're still so that you can become more aware of how your mind works.

Your mind is running you at all times to the point that you're often unaware of what your brain is telling you to do. Meditation is an important act of self-care because it helps you communicate with your mind and understand some of your own drives and motivations. It's only in silent introspection that you can hear the story or narrative your mind is telling you.

A meditation practice will help you understand your own motivations, programming, and desires to stay centered, stable, and clear-headed.

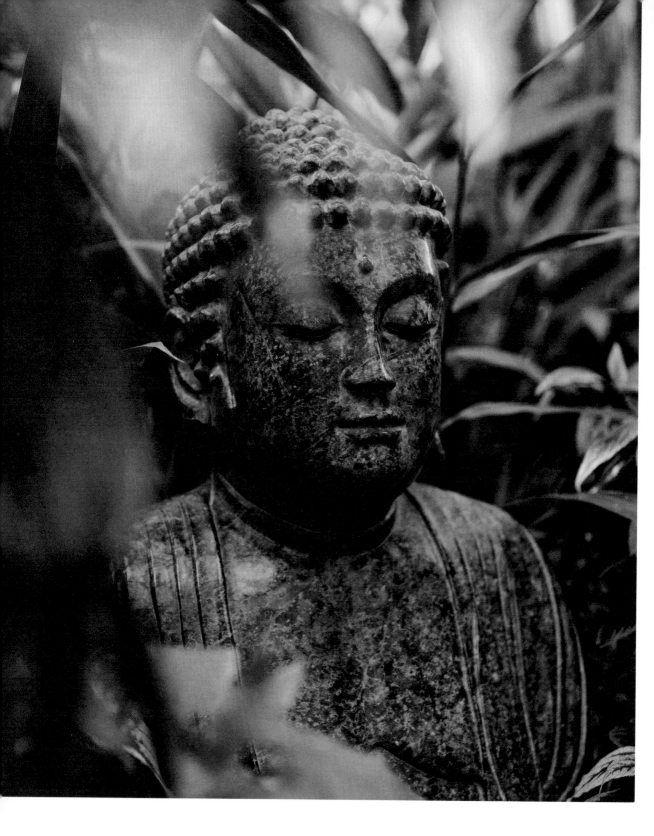

Learn to Meditate in Five Minutes

This exercise helps break down meditation so that it's accessible and achievable. During the first five minutes of your meditation practice:

(1) Find a comfortable sitting position: on the floor, on a mat, on the grass, or in a chair.

(2) Close your eyes and sit in silence.

(3) Breathe in through your nose and exhale through your mouth. Track your breath. This just means being conscious of the breath entering and leaving your body.

(4) As you track your breath, you'll notice that things become a little more "still."

(5) If a thought enters your mind while you're in stillness, acknowledge the thought, make note of it, and then let it pass.

(6) To refocus yourself, return to your breathing. Fill yourself with air through your nose and mouth. Do this each time a thought arises and then go back to your breath to center yourself.

(7) Practice this for five minutes. As you continue your practice (each morning is ideal!), you can increase the amount of time you remain in meditation.

Chakras and Unblocking Them

Think of chakras as the major centers of energy within your body. The belief around chakras is that all seven chakras should be "open" to promote harmony and balance in your system. The concept of a "blocked chakra" is that if one of your primary energy centers in your body is blocked. Then the whole system is off balance and the chakra needs to be cleared.

Each chakra is correlated with a different place in your body and has its own specific meaning and color. You can incorporate the color and/or crystals[30] associated with a chakra to help unblock it.[31]

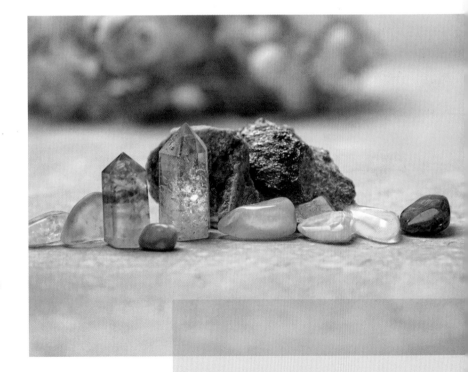

① THE ROOT CHAKRA

Color: *Red*
Crystals: *Hematite, Smoky Quartz, Red Jasper*

This chakra is at the base of your spine near your tailbone, and it represents your foundation. When the root chakra is open, you feel grounded, stable, and authentic. Feeling unstable, dealing with basic survival issues like food and money, anxiety, and an inability to trust are indications that this chakra is blocked.

To unblock your root chakra, practice grounding (page 29) or utilize the yoga tree pose (page 19).

② THE SACRAL CHAKRA

Color: *Orange*
Crystals: *Carnelian, Tiger's Eye, Orange Calcite*

The sacral chakra is located two inches below your belly button. It represents how you deal with emotions—both your own and those of others. When this chakra is open, you feel in tune with your sexuality, connected to creativity and pleasure. This chakra may be blocked if you're experiencing pelvic pain, sexual blocks, or difficulty in your intimate relationships.

To unblock your sacral chakra, practice meditating in silence for long periods of time to reconnect with yourself. Meditation is covered earlier in this section of the book (page 142).

③ THE SOLAR PLEXUS CHAKRA

Color: *Yellow*
Crystals: *Pyrite, Yellow Jasper, Citrine*

The solar plexus chakra is located in your upper abdomen, which is the area where your gut instinct or the feeling of butterflies in your stomach comes into play. This is also where your ego and sense of self reside. When this chakra is open, you feel confident in your life and have positive self-esteem. This chakra may be blocked if you're experiencing digestive issues or feelings of judgment.

To unblock your solar plexus chakra, scream! Seriously. Scream at least three times in a row.[32] If you need to scream more, do so. This helps release the blocked energy.

④ THE HEART CHAKRA

Color: *Green*
Crystals: *Rose Quartz, Rhodonite, Aventurine*

This chakra is located in the center of your chest near your heart. When this chakra is open, you're able to give and receive love and live with courage. But when it's blocked, you might have an aversion to love, an inability to accept love, a lack of compassion, or feelings of rejection.

To unblock your heart chakra, write yourself a love letter (page 83).

⑤ THE THROAT CHAKRA

Color: *Blue*
Crystals: *Aquamarine, Sodalite, Angelite*

This chakra has a self-explanatory location: it's located in your throat. The throat chakra is connected with expression. When this chakra is open, you're better able to communicate clearly and honestly. Your throat chakra may be blocked if you feel guilty, misunderstood, or unable to manifest the things you want in your life.

To unblock your throat chakra, repeat your favorite affirmation confidently for ten seconds. This is covered in Section 3 (page 118).

⑥ THE THIRD EYE CHAKRA

Color: *Indigo*
Crystals: *Amethyst, Fluorite, Angelite*

This chakra, also known as the "eye of the soul," is located between your eyebrows. When the third eye chakra is open, you feel connected to your intuition. You may also feel more imaginative and like you've reached a higher level of wisdom. This chakra may be blocked if you're experiencing headaches or nightmares, struggling with making concrete decisions, have a hormonal imbalance, or can't express feelings of empathy.

To unblock your third eye chakra, keep a dream journal.[33] Keep a journal next to your bed and jot down your dreams, or nightmares, when you wake up.

⑦ THE CROWN CHAKRA

Color: *Violet*
Crystals: *Amethyst, Clear Quartz, Moonstone*

This chakra is located at the highest point of your body on the very top of your head. When you reach a point of openness with this chakra, you can access a higher consciousness. This is all about being fully connected spiritually while existing on a physical plane. The crown chakra is also connected to your inner and outer beauty. This chakra may be blocked if you're experiencing insomnia, isolation, or depression.

To unblock your crown chakra, connect with others and get outside of yourself. Try volunteering, a topic covered in Section 5 (page 157).

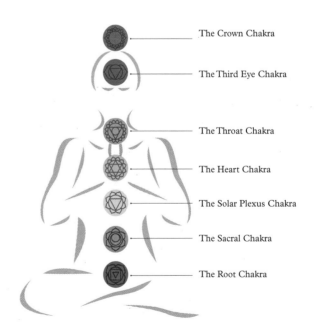

The Crown Chakra

The Third Eye Chakra

The Throat Chakra

The Heart Chakra

The Solar Plexus Chakra

The Sacral Chakra

The Root Chakra

Manifestation

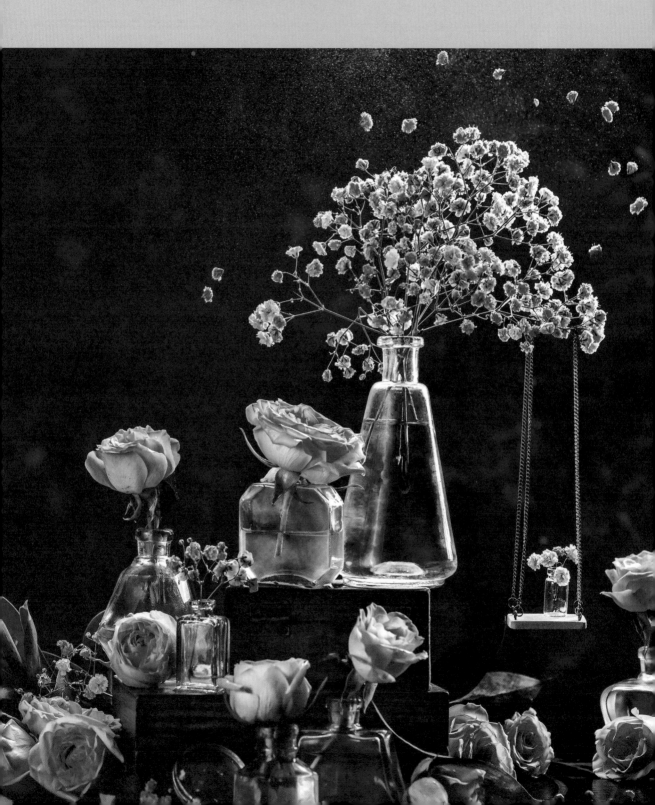

Manifestation is using your energy, belief system, thoughts, and visualization to bring something into your physical reality. In practice, the steps of manifestation could look like this:

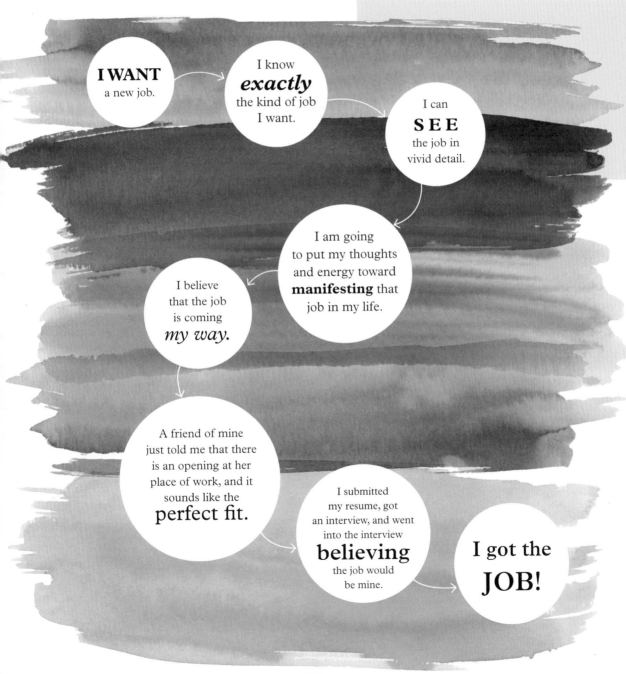

I **WANT** a new job.

I know *exactly* the kind of job I want.

I can **SEE** the job in vivid detail.

I am going to put my thoughts and energy toward **manifesting** that job in my life.

I believe that the job is coming *my way.*

A friend of mine just told me that there is an opening at her place of work, and it sounds like the **perfect fit.**

I submitted my resume, got an interview, and went into the interview **believing** the job would be mine.

I got the **JOB!**

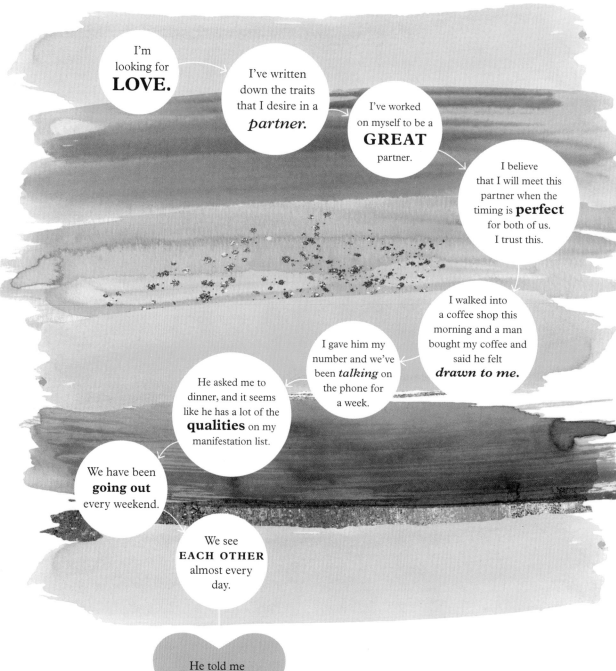

I'm looking for **LOVE.**

I've written down the traits that I desire in a *partner*.

I've worked on myself to be a **GREAT** partner.

I believe that I will meet this partner when the timing is **perfect** for both of us. I trust this.

I walked into a coffee shop this morning and a man bought my coffee and said he felt *drawn to me.*

I gave him my number and we've been *talking* on the phone for a week.

He asked me to dinner, and it seems like he has a lot of the **qualities** on my manifestation list.

We have been **going out** every weekend.

We see **EACH OTHER** almost every day.

He told me **he loves me!** And I love him!

Essentially, manifestation is a *specific* vision that's fueled by positive energy—a powerful combination that can turn your dreams into a reality.

Practicing Manifestation

Decide on something specific you *really want* and *believe* that you can manifest. Focus on something you deeply want that resonates with your gut instinct and somehow serves the greater good.[34]

For a manifestation to appear, you need to get rid of your blocks. A negative mindset can block a manifestation. Do mindset work first so that you're coming from a place of positivity, confidence, and belief. Make sure any toxic people—those who criticize, doubt, belittle, or negatively impact you—are removed from your life, or at least establish boundaries to limit your interaction and stop their impact. You also need to assess the timing of your request. If you want to manifest writing a blockbuster screenplay, it's not going to happen tomorrow; you need ample time to write it. Be realistic with the timing of your manifestation.

Be incredibly specific about your visualization. When you think about what you want to manifest, be specific, down to the tiniest detail. Close your eyes and sit in silence. Meditate if you need to clear your headspace. Imagine your manifestation in vivid detail and using all of your senses. Imagine how you will feel when your manifestation occurs. Make it as real as you can in your mind's eye. Remember you don't need to know how it will manifest—you just need to trust that it will. Bonus points: after you visualize it, write down every tiny detail. Then put this paper in a place you look at every day to give continual positive energy and belief to your manifestation.

Don't act unless you feel—in your gut—that you're supposed to do something. The aforementioned three steps are typically all the action you need to take. However, if you feel your gut instinct positively telling you to do something (and it's not driven by anxiety, doubt, or worry), then you should respond with action.

Once your manifestation appears, express gratitude and appreciate what you have. As you continue to manifest in the future, you want to have a good track record of recognizing what you have been given in the past. Gratitude is so important. If you're keeping a gratitude journal (page 81), this is a good place to write down how grateful you are for what has already come your way. You can also say "thank you" out loud or consciously celebrate what you have in your life.

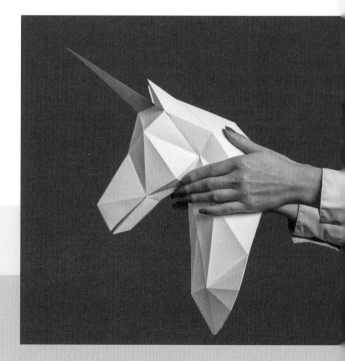

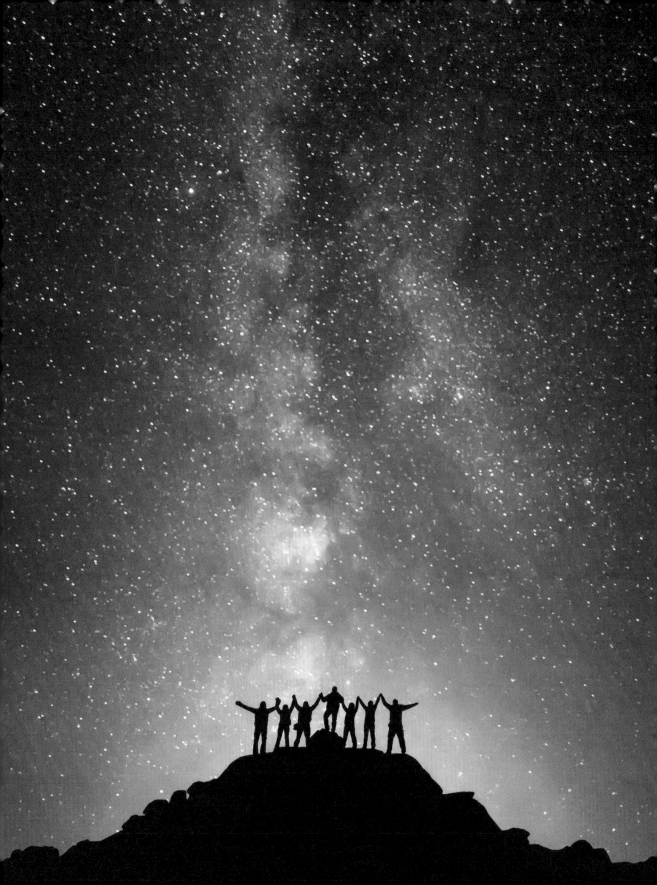

5

SOCIAL SELF-CARE

"There are rare people who will show up at the right time, help you through the hard times and stay into your best times... those are the keepers."

—NAUSICAA TWILA

People

Although much of this book focuses on things you may do alone in the name of self-care, connecting with other individuals and the world around you is also an imperative part of the process. As you grow into a more complete, focused, clear, happy, and centered version of yourself, it's necessary that you share this positivity with others.

The ripple effect, essentially when you drop a rock into a pond and it sends out numerous ripples around it, is real. You are the rock. Drop yourself into the world with your self-care cup full to the brim and watch the impact your energy has on the environment and individuals around you.

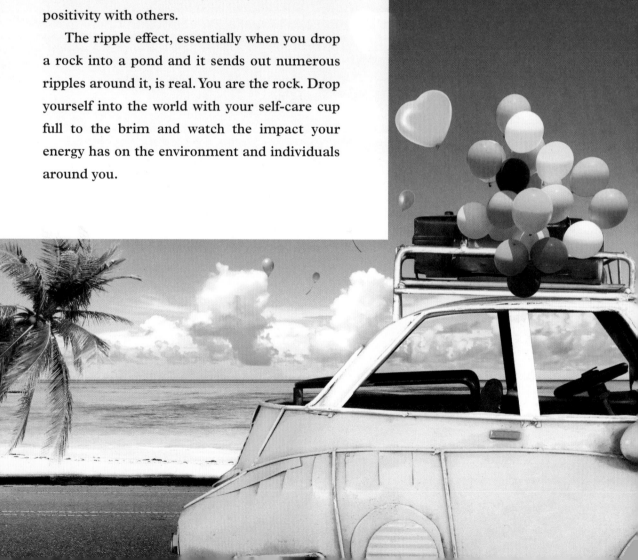

Friendship Assessment

Friendship is powerful. At its best, it can build you up, provide you with a sense of love and community, increase the amount of fun you experience, and create a reliable support system. At its worst—if the friends you choose are toxic—it can be destructive, lead you away from your value system, and negatively impact the trajectory of your life.

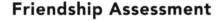

To quickly identify if your friendship is a healthy one that enhances your life, ask yourself the following:

After you spend quality time with this friend, do you:

1. Feel more energized and positive about life?

2. Feel drained, exhausted, and negative about life?

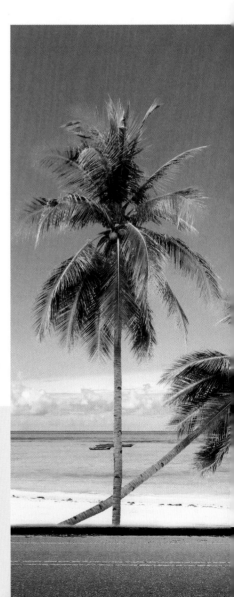

If your answer was number one, nourish this healthy friendship. If the answer is number two, it's best for both parties involved to part ways.

As you age, you may find that you become more selective with your friendships. Part of this is because getting older tends to have a host of responsibilities attached to it that decrease the amount of free time you have, which limits the amount of people you can prioritize. Another element of this is maturity; as you begin to know yourself more deeply, it becomes clear which friends fit within your value system and desires and which fall outside of your spectrum.

To give you a simple visual, think of your closet. When you were younger you probably gathered a variety of clothing based on convenience, low cost, or items that were given to you. But as you got older, chances are you realized that some of this clothing was poor quality, not the right fit for you, didn't go with the rest of your wardrobe, or no longer fit your personality or style. As you identify your style, you tend to purchase fewer clothes of higher quality, shop with intention, and learn to identify the gaps in your wardrobe that needs to be filled.

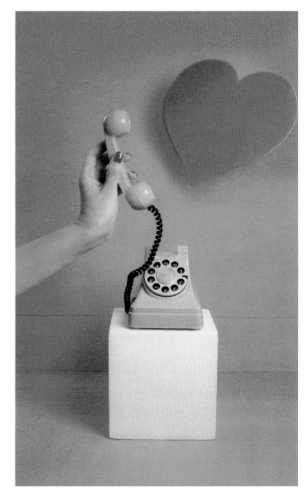

With time and experience, you're able to discern the difference between the items that are keepers and which ones don't fit or serve you anymore. This is a lot like friends. Using the second question above, assess your "friend closet" once a year—just like you would do with your clothes closet—and remove any individuals who no longer fit in with the trajectory of your life.

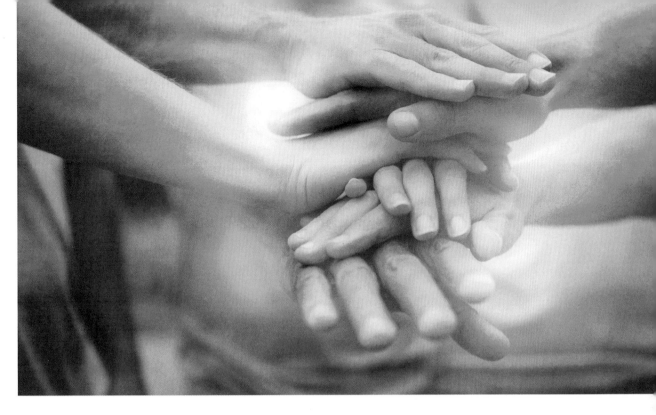

Volunteering

Though volunteering appears to be a wholly selfless act, it's also beneficial to you and your self-care. There are a myriad of perks to volunteering, including:[35]

- You can meet like-minded people and connect with people you may have not encountered otherwise.

- It helps diminish stress, anxiety, and even anger.

- It can combat depression and ultimately bring you happiness; being helpful to others has been proven to make people feel a sense of pleasure.

- Volunteering provides a sense of purpose and fulfillment.

- Volunteering can be really fun.

When choosing where and how you want to volunteer, start by looking at your own interests.

- Do you love to read? Consider reading to children after school or to sight-impaired adults.

- Do you love athletics? Work with a local facility that takes in teens and help facilitate a league. Or you can volunteer for the Special Olympics.

- Do you love being outside? Help at a community garden.

- Do you love teaching? Teach at a local women's shelter or to a group of at-risk teens.

- Do you love animals? Your local animal shelter may be looking for onsite assistance or foster families.

Once you choose your cause, volunteer once a month for consistency. If you really love it, you might find yourself volunteering weekly, or more!

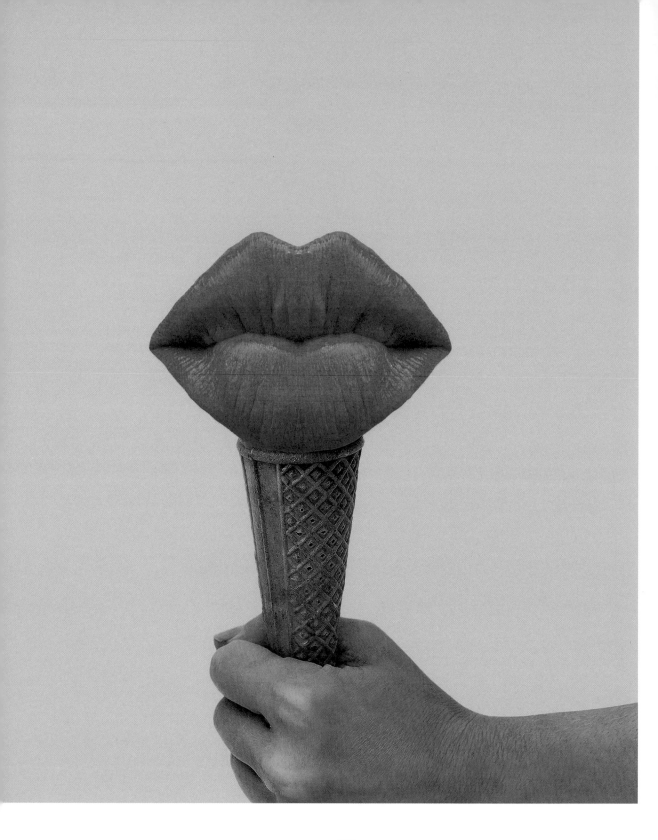

Ask for Help

Sometimes regardless of the amount of self-care you pour into yourself, you can't do everything alone. Asking for help is not a weakness—it's a strength in that you recognize your present limitations and are willing to be vulnerable.

There are many places to go for help, both personal and professional. These include:

- **Friends:** Reach out to a trusted friend if you need assistance or a connection. Most people don't know that you need them—or what you need—if you don't specifically tell them. Don't be afraid to ask for exactly what you need during a difficult time.

- **Family:** If you have a healthy family dynamic, this can be a good place to go for support because you will be loved, not judged. Reach out to a professional if you don't have unconditional family support.

- **Professional Help:** Therapists and counselors have the ability to listen without judgment and can help you see things from a different perspective. They can be a wonderful source of clarity, and it can feel freeing to be able to talk to someone who is thoroughly trained to help you.

- **Religious Counseling:** If you have a specific religious affiliation, you may find it beneficial to seek assistance through your religious institution. This way your belief system and faith can be woven into your road to optimal self-improvement.

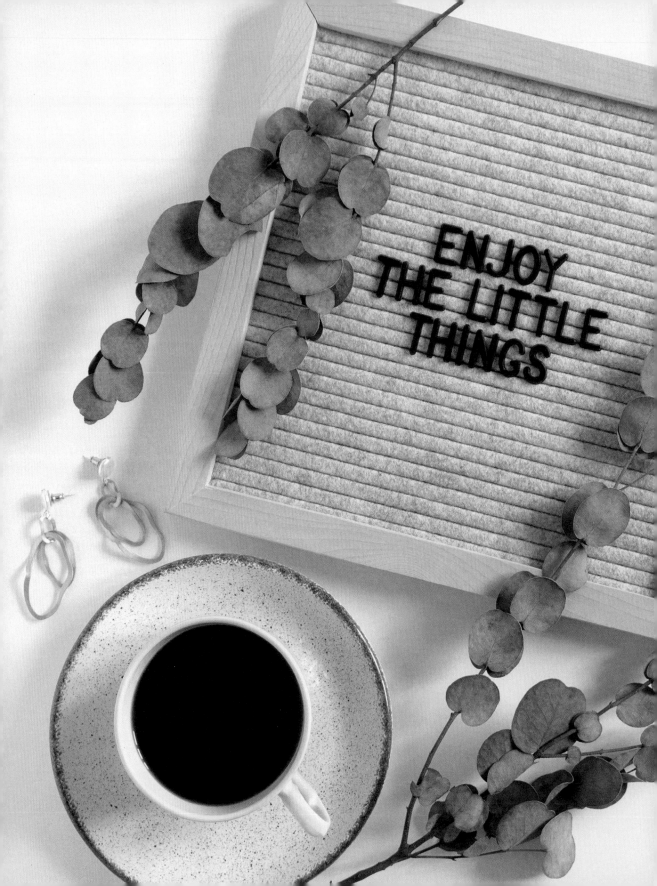

Stay in Touch

I feel strongly about being part of a community that's committed to self-care and supports and encourages one another along the self-care journey—and I'd love to stay in contact with you!

If you'd like to connect with me, you can find me on Instagram:

@blonderambitions

If this book resonated with you, I would be honored if you would share it on social media! Please use the hashtag:

#thecompleteguidetoselfcare

I have an extensive background in speaking at conventions, symposiums, retreats, workshops, on podcasts, and online. If you'd like to book a speaking engagement, please email me at:

blonderambitions.kiki@gmail.com

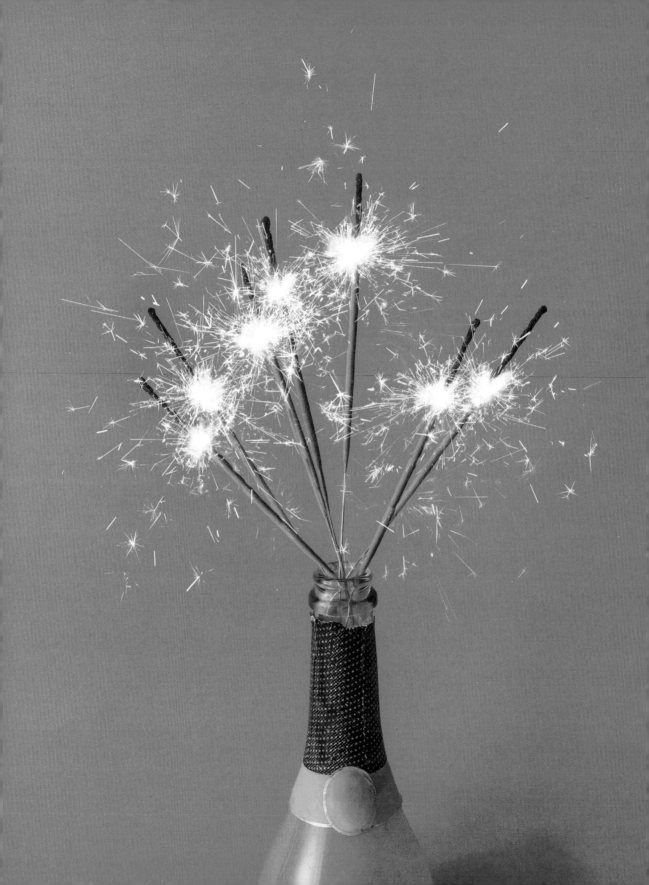

Thank You & Acknowledgments

To my father and brother who taught me
so much about intellectual and physical self-care.

To my mother and sister who taught me
endless amounts about emotional self-care.

To my friends who taught me
about social self-care.

And to God, the ultimate light, who
taught me about spiritual self-care.

To all of you for choosing to honor yourselves.

Finally, to myself for choosing me!
Learning to love myself. Sharing the journey.
Connecting with a higher frequency.
Choosing to live in light every single day.

Here's to driving our ship straight through the
storm with a glint in our eye knowing that we can
surely make it through because—even without
the stars to guide us—we have memorized their
location right behind the clouds... and a knowing
that they will look brighter than they ever have
when we get to the other side.

Rise, woman, rise.

INDEX

RESOURCES

1 "Does Walking Barefoot have Health Benefits?" *Healthline,* 2018, https://www.healthline.com/health/walking-barefoot.

2 "Never Had a Massage? What You Should Know." *Mayo Clinic,* Mayo Foundation for Medical Education and Research, 6 Oct. 2018, www.mayoclinic.org/healthy-lifestyle/stress-management/in-depth/massage/art-20045743.

3 Editors, *Reader's Digest.* "Heal Yourself: 17 Tricks for a Soothing Self-Massage." *The Healthy,* www.thehealthy.com/home-remedies/self-massage/.

4 + 5 Legg, Timothy J and Nall, Rachel. "What Are the Benefits of Sunlight?" May 25, 2018. https://www.healthline.com/health/depression/benefits-sunlight.

6 + 7 McIntosh, James. "15 Benefits of Drinking Water and Other Water Facts." *Medical News Today,* MediLexicon International, 16 July 2018, www.medicalnewstoday.com/articles/290814.php.

8 Jennings, Kerri-Anne. "A Quick Guide to Intuitive Eating" June 25, 2019. https://www.healthline.com/nutrition/quick-guide-intuitive-eating#basics

9 Nordqvist, Joseph. "Apples: Health Benefits, Facts, Research." *Medical News Today,* MediLexicon International, 11 Apr. 2017, www.medicalnewstoday.com/articles/267290.php.

10 Gunnars, Kris. "12 Proven Health Benefits of Avocado" June 29, 2018. https://www.healthline.com/nutrition/12-proven-benefits-of-avocado#section5

11 "Bananas: A Nutritional Powerhouse." *WebMD,* WebMD, www.webmd.com/food-recipes/health-benefits-bananas.

12 Link, Rachel, "7 Health Benefits of Eating Cucumber" May 19, 2017. https://www.healthline.com/nutrition/7-health-benefits-of-cucumber.

13 "What Do Face Rollers Actually Do for Your Skin?" *Girlboss,* 20 Sept. 2018, www.girlboss.com/beauty/face-rollers-benefits.

14 Boone, DaMonica, and Hannah Baxter. "How to Use a Jade Roller." *Coveteur,* Coveteur, 2 Dec. 2018, coveteur.com/2018/11/28/how-to-use-jade-roller-depuff-face/.

15 Taylor, et al. "The Amazing Benefits of Argan Oil for Hair and Skin." *The Crunchy Moose,* 25 June 2018, thecrunchymoose.com/argan-oil-2/.

16 Nordqvist, Joseph. "Lavender: Health Benefits and Uses." *Medical News Today,* MediLexicon International, 4 Mar. 2019, www.medicalnewstoday.com/articles/265922.php#benefits.

17 Cobb, Cynthia. "How Does Tea Tree Oil Help the Skin?" May 2, 2018. https://www.healthline.com/health/tea-tree-oil-for-skin#benefits-and-uses

18 Patulny, Lisa. "13 Reasons Why You Should Be Using Jojoba Oil Every Day." *Byrdie,* Byrdie, 18 June 2019, www.byrdie.com/jojoba-oil-beauty-uses.

19 "How Many Hours of Sleep Do You Need?" *Mayo Clinic,* Mayo Foundation for Medical Education and Research, 6 June 2019, www.mayoclinic.org/healthy-lifestyle/adult-health/expert-answers/how-many-hours-of-sleep-are-enough/faq-20057898.

20 Stibich, Mark. "10 Top Health Benefits of Sleep." *Verywell Health,* Verywell Health, 5 Sept. 2019, www.verywellhealth.com/top-health-benefits-of-a-good-nights-sleep-2223766.

21 Legg, Timothy J and Nall, Rachel. "What Are the Benefits of Sunlight?" May 25, 2018. https://www.healthline.com/health/depression/benefits-sunlight.

22 "Circadian Rhythms." *National Institute of General Medical Sciences,* U.S. Department of Health and Human Services, www.nigms.nih.gov/education/pages/factsheet_circadianrhythms.aspx.

23 Harvard Health Publishing. "Blue Light Has a Dark Side." *Harvard Health,* www.health.harvard.edu/staying-healthy/blue-light-has-a-dark-side.

24 "Sleeping Tips & Tricks." *National Sleep Foundation*, www.sleepfoundation.org/articles/healthy-sleep-tips.

25 Pfizer Medical Team. "10 Health Benefits of Music." *Get Healthy Stay Healthy*, www.gethealthystayhealthy.com/articles/10-health-benefits-of-music.

26 S., Christopher. "The 5 Easiest Instruments Perfect for Adult Learners." TakeLessons Blog, Christopher S. Https://Tl-Cdn.s3.Amazonaws.com/Images/LogoTagline.svg, 15 Dec. 2018, takelessons.com/blog/easiest-instrument-for-adults.

27 Winter, Catherine. "10 Benefits of Reading: Why You Should Read Every Day." *Lifehack*, Lifehack, 4 June 2019, www.lifehack.org/articles/lifestyle/10-benefits-reading-why-you-should-read-everyday.html.

28 "6 Benefits of an Uncluttered Space." *Psychology Today*, Sussex Publishers, www.psychologytoday.com/us/blog/in-practice/201802/6-benefits-uncluttered-space.

29 Kim, Larry. "Multitasking Is Killing Your Brain." *Medium*, The Startup, 30 Apr. 2018, medium.com/swlh/multitasking-is-killing-your-brain-cca83edca7bb.

30 Kim, Larry. "Multitasking Is Killing Your Brain." *Medium*, The Startup, 30 Apr. 2018, medium.com/swlh/multitasking-is-killing-your-brain-cca83edca7bb.

31 Lee, Joel. "How to Do a Social Media Detox (and Why You Should Right Away)." *MakeUseOf*, 24 Mar. 2017, www.makeuseof.com/tag/social-media-detox/.

32 Heatheraskinosiemuse. "What Are the 7 Chakras in Your Body?: Chakras Meanings." *Energy Muse Blog*, 15 May 2019, www.energymuse.com/blog/chakra-stones-chart-chakra-awareness/.

33 Cameron, Yogi. "A Beginner's Guide to the 7 Chakras." *Mindbodygreen*, Mindbodygreen, 10 Sept. 2019, www.mindbodygreen.com/0-91/The-7-Chakras-for-Beginners.html.

34 Matluck, Erica, and N.p. "A Simple Exercise to Unblock Your Chakras." *Mindbodygreen*, Mindbodygreen, 23 Aug. 2019, www.mindbodygreen.com/0-9921/a-simple-exercise-to-unblock-your-chakras.html.

35 Matluck, Erica, and N.p. "A Simple Exercise to Unblock Your Chakras." *Mindbodygreen*, Mindbodygreen, 23 Aug. 2019, www.mindbodygreen.com/0-9921/a-simple-exercise-to-unblock-your-chakras.html.

36 Hurst, Katherine. "Manifestation Guide: How to Manifest Anything You Want In 24hrs." *The Law of Attraction*, 31 May 2019, www.thelawofattraction.com/manifest-something-want-24hrs-less/.

37 "Volunteering and Its Surprising Benefits." *HelpGuide.org*, 16 July 2019, www.helpguide.org/articles/healthy-living/volunteering-and-its-surprising-benefits.htm.

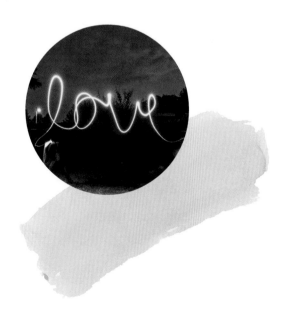

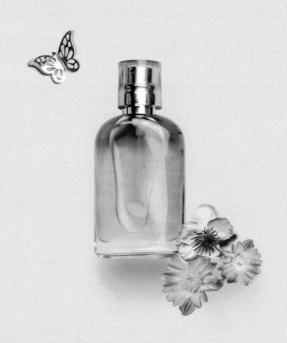